cf
39.95

D1592473

WITHDRAWN

Treating Alcohol and Drug Abuse in the Elderly

Anne M. Gurnack, MSW, PhD, is the senior editor for this volume and is Professor and Chair of the Political Science Department at the University of Wisconsin-Parkside. Her interests include public health policy, social gerontology, and public administration. She has published numerous works in the area of elderly alcohol and drug misuse, and was editor of the previous volume on this topic published by Springer in 1997: *Older Adults' Misuse of Alcohol, Medicines, and Other Drugs: Research and Practice Issues.* Her current articles focus on alcohol and drug problems of elderly American ethnic groups.

Roland M. Atkinson, MD, is Professor of Psychiatry at the School of Medicine, Oregon Health and Science University (OHSU). Dr. Atkinson received his medical and psychiatric training at Stanford and UCLA Schools of Medicine, and studied geriatric psychiatry at the Maudsley Hospital, London. He has been on the faculty at OHSU since 1976 and was also Chief of Psychiatry at the Veterans Affairs Medical Center in Portland for 15 years. He has studied alcohol problems in the geriatric population since 1982.

Nancy J. Osgood, PhD, is a Professor in the Department of Gerontology at Virginia Commonwealth University. Her interests include suicide in the elderly, geriatric alcoholism, and depression. She is the author of *Alcoholism and aging: An annotated bibliography and review* (1995, Westport, CT: Greenwood Press). She was the principal investigator for the project, *A Detection and Prevention Program for Geriatric Alcoholism,* funded by the Administration on Aging.

Treating Alcohol and Drug Abuse in the Elderly

Anne M. Gurnack, *MSW, PhD*
Roland Atkinson, *MD*
Nancy J. Osgood, *PhD, Editors*

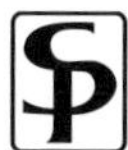 *Springer Publishing Company*

Copyright © 2002 by Springer Publishing Company, Inc.

All rights reserved

No part of this publication may be reproduced, stored in a retrieval system, or transmitted in any form or by any means, electronic, mechanical, photocopying, recording, or otherwise, without the prior permission of Springer Publishing Company, Inc.

Springer Publishing Company, Inc.
536 Broadway
New York, NY 10012-3955

Acquisitions Editor: Sheri W. Sussman
Production Editor: Sara Yoo
Cover design by Susan Hauley

01 02 03 04 05 / 5 4 3 2 1

Library of Congress Cataloging-in-Publication-Data

Treating alcohol and drug abuse in the elderly / Anne M. Gurnack,
Roland M. Atkinson, Nancy J. Osgood, editors.
p. cm.
Includes bibliographical references and index.
ISBN 0-8261-1434-2
1. Aged—Alcohol use. 2. Aged—Drug use. 3. Alcoholism—Treatment.
4. Medication abuse—Treatment. I. Gurnack, Anne Marie. II. Atkinson, Roland M., 1936– . III. Osgood, Nancy J.
HV5138.T74 2001
362.292'8'0846—dc21

2001049097

Printed in the United States of America by Maple-Vail.

Contents

Part III: Other Addictive Problems

Contributors

Wendy L. Adams, MD, MPH
University of Nebraska Medical Center
Omaha, Nebraska

Neal R. Boyd, EdD, MSPH
The George Washington University Medical Center
Reston, Virginia

Constance L. Coogle, PhD
Virginia Center on Aging
Virginia Commonwealth University
Richmond, Virginia

Larry W. Dupree, PhD
Department of Aging and Mental Health
The Florida Mental Health Institute
University of South Florida
Tampa, Florida

Richard E. Finlayson, MD
Mayo Clinic and Mayo Foundation
Rochester, Minnesota

Michael F. Fleming, MD, MPH
Department of Family Medicine
University of Wisconsin
Madison, Wisconsin

Virginia E. Hofmann, MD
Mayo Clinic and Mayo Foundation
Rochester, Minnesota

Rita Holden, RN
Department of Psychiatry
University of Pennsylvania
Philadelphia, Pennsylvania

Sahana Misra, MD
Oregon Health Services University
Portland, Oregon

George E. Murphy, MD
Washington University
St. Louis, Missouri

C. Tracy Orleans, PhD
Robert Wood Johnson Foundation
Princeton, New Jersey

David W. Oslin, MD
Department of Psychiatry
University of Pennsylvania
Philadelphia, Pennsylvania

Ronald M. Pavalko, PhD
University of Wisconsin-Parkside
Kenosha, Wisconsin

Lawrence Schonfeld, PhD
Department of Aging and Mental Health
The Florida Mental Health Institute
University of South Florida
Tampa, Florida

Preface

We are excited about the final arrival of this much anticipated book about the treatment of problems of elderly alcohol and drug misuse. This project was a long labor of love for all three of us. We therefore are grateful to our families and loved ones who tolerated us during the four years devoted to the preparation of this manuscript. We totally underestimated the effort that was needed to produce a modern, "state of the art," clinically oriented volume. But we are very pleased with the final product.

First, we are happy to acknowledge the monumental efforts of our outstanding contributors who were willing to revise and revise and revise their chapters. As you will see, the chapters contained here are the best these wonderful professionals could produce.

The time contributed by the UW Parkside library staff was invaluable, particularly by Cindy Bryan. They went to great lengths to ensure the accuracy of the numerous citations contained in this book.

We would also like to thank the many outside reviewers who critically analyzed these chapters throughout the entire development and production process.

Finally, we give hearty thanks to the staff of Springer Publishing who always insist on high-quality manuscripts.

Anne M. Gurnack
Roland M. Atkinson
Nancy J. Osgood

1

Introduction and Overview

Anne M. Gurnack

During the last decade scholarship has increased severalfold in the area of aging and substance misuse. We are amazed to see this continuing interest in a subject that was neglected previously. As our population continues to age and elders' use of prescribed medications, alcohol, and various drugs increases, we anticipate that more elderly will have problems with these substances in the future.

The types of substances that are being used or misused may change as various cohorts like "baby boomers" mature into old age. At the present time there are two major categories on which most scholars focus. These categories are alcohol and prescription medication misuse. These two categories are very different in nature.

Health care professionals and researchers have acknowledged that older problem drinkers are hard to identify and often remain a hidden population. They are rarely admitted to traditional addiction treatments. As early as the late 1960s and continuing on through the mid-1970s, the published literature related to alcohol misuse and aging very often was made up of speculations about the prevalence of the problem and the results of community-based surveys or evaluations of treatment programs. During the last 20 years, studies have described pilot treatment programs and treatment differences between older and younger drinkers. Also, researchers have identified alternative case-finding methods focusing on programs within aging services, emergency medical care, general hospital populations, veterans hospitals, gate-keeper programs, and retirement communities.

But unlike alcohol abuse, most elderly medication misuse is thought of as unintentional, as a result of failure to understand and subsequent noncompliance with prescription instructions by the physician, adverse side effects, and prescribing practices by professionals. Most programs focus on the abuse of alcohol, and the identification of this related problem creates many challenges for professionals. Again this situation may change in the near future as the present baby boomer generation matures and demonstrates more complex addictive patterns. For this reason this volume also includes some attention to tobacco and gambling addictions, which are receiving attention in this modern approach to understanding these very often interdependent problems.

During the last two decades publications have focused mainly on the empirical aspects of these subjects. The first volume printed by Springer Publishing in 1997, for the most part addressed research issues of elderly alcohol and drug misuse (Gurnack, 1997). In fact, as a result of this publication, health care professionals demanded more practical treatment-oriented information. We are therefore very excited about offering this type of information to the practitioner who must deal with elderly use of alcohol and drugs on a daily basis.

The articles which follow were prepared by an internationally known team of scholars and practitioners in the field of elderly alcohol and drug misuse. Therefore, the material presented in this book is "state of the art" and intended to guide the beginning practitioner through the process of understanding and applying the knowledge gained so far in the area of elderly alcohol and drug misuse.

The book is divided into three parts. The first set of chapters introduces material related to assessment and screening for alcohol and drugs and discusses several of the complications which may arise from these conditions, such as depression and possible suicide.

The second part looks at the various treatment approaches available for older adults who misuse alcohol and drugs. Case examples are included in all chapters and provide a guide for those who are just beginning the study of these issues. And for those practitioners who are very knowledgeable with this population, the material will reinforce the "best practices" developed through the years by those with extensive "hands-on" experience.

The third part addresses issues of tobacco and gambling addiction, both of which are often related to elderly alcohol and drug misuse. Similar patterns of addiction are often identified in these related disorders.

The final chapter addresses prevention and reflects a very new emphasis. The authors describe a model that exists in Virginia as well as provide valuable information on prevention of elderly alcohol and substance misuse.

Recognition, Assessment, and Complications of Elderly Alcohol and Drug Misuse

The first chapter in this section by Oslin covers various tools of screening those elders who may be misusing alcohol and other substances, such as the geriatric version of the Short Michigan Alcohol Screening Test (SMAST-G).

But perhaps more important, the author delineates carefully a number of categories of drinking which should be addressed within the context of the screening and assessment process. These groups include: At-Risk Use, At-Risk Alcohol Use, At-Risk Benzodiazepine or Other Prescription Use, Problem Use, and Substance Dependence. Assessment and recognition is related to these categories.

"At Risk Use" is defined as consumption above a specified level that may or may not meet criteria for abuse or dependence. The author states that the purpose of defining a group of individuals who meet this definition of a target pattern of use is to identify a population that is at high risk of developing problems related to alcohol or medication use and then intervene in a preventive manner.

"At-Risk Alcohol Use" is defined as more than seven standard drinks per week. This level of drinking was determined by a nationally recognized panel of experts. In contrast, "At-Risk Benzodiazepine or Other Prescription Medication Use" is harder to define. The problem here is that patients may be on multiple medications in combination with over-the-counter drugs often resulting in complications.

"Problem Use" has a clearer definition and is said to be the consumption of alcohol or the use of medications or drugs that has already led to at least one definable problem or consequence. And finally, "Substance Dependence" is currently defined in the Diagnostic and Statistical Manual Fourth Edition (DSM–IV) and is outlined in this chapter. Dr. Oslin carefully illustrates these categories and screening/assessment to case studies which are found throughout the chapter.

In the second contribution, Adams looks at the effects of alcohol on medical illnesses and medication interactions. Her excellent case illustrations demonstrate that alcohol and medications may be linked to virtually all body systems. She states that alcoholic liver disease is the most widely recognized medical complication of alcoholism, but serious damage can also occur to the nervous system, the cardiovascular system, the gastrointestinal system, and bone and muscle damage can occur as well. And the risk of some cancers is increased among heavy drinkers.

Other health conditions identified by Adams include osteoporosis and possible medication interactions. Alcohol, she states, is used concurrently with medications by a large number of elderly people. And it is important for health care professionals to ask patients about their alcohol and medication use when it puts them at risk for health problems.

In addition to physical health effects, the next chapter by Atkinson looks at the association of alcohol-related problems with other psychiatric disorders. In fact he cites studies which find that as much as 50% of alcoholics in every age group had additional "comorbid" mental disorders. Such mental disorders may include depression. The author includes some very insightful case examples which differentiate between depression that is related to alcohol use and depression that is a separate and distinct disorder. The health care professional is therefore given the tools by which to distinguish these conditions. For example, there is a section which relates to treating depression in patients who continue to drink. He raises the question of whether antidepressants should be continued to be prescribed to those patients who continue to drink.

The Atkinson work also focuses on other conditions such as cognitive impairment and dementia related to drinking. The final condition of anxiety is examined again as a disorder associated with the consumption of alcohol or one which may persist as a separate comorbid condition.

Finally, the chapter addresses comorbid drug use such as tobacco, cocaine, and other substances. The author concludes with some insightful comments about assessment and treatment of these patients with comorbid mental disorders.

The final chapter of this section focuses on a very serious issue, i.e., that of alcoholism, drug abuse, and suicide in the elderly. Murphy's contribution is a concise, beautifully crafted analysis of this profound concern. He enumerates a series of risk factors for suicide in substance abusers which include: continued substance abuse; expressed suicidal thoughts and attempts; little social support available; concurrent depression; poor physical health; loss or lack of employment; and living alone.

Dr. Murphy emphasizes the need for health care professionals to engage in efforts to prevent suicide. First, he says one must engage in diagnosis. Next, the level of suicide risk must be assessed. And, third, appropriate treatment approaches must be applied, such as pharmcotherapy or psychotherapy. However, one must be cautious because unless one is trained and skilled in the use of psychotherapies, pharmacotherapy is the better choice.

Treatment of Alcohol Use Disorders

This lead chapter of Part Two presents an excellent overview of treatment strategies. As Dr. Fleming points out, the alcohol treatment field is moving toward a new public health paradigm, that is, one which focuses on reducing alcohol use to low-risk levels. This approach allows the health care professional to serve a larger percentage of the elderly population who misuse alcohol rather than those who meet the criteria for alcoholism.

Fleming outlines the components of brief intervention and treatment of alcohol problems. The steps in this process are as follows: assessment; direct feedback; contract negotiating and goal setting; behavioral modification techniques; self-help bibliotherapy; and follow-up reinforcement.

In addition, he outlines a series of stages through which the patient may pass on the way to treatment. This model helps the professional to understand that there are varying states of awareness for the patient and that he can help guide them and motivate them to change. These stages are illustrated profusely throughout the text by the inclusion of summary tables.

The brief intervention model presented in this chapter presents an interesting and useful tool that can be used by a primary care physician. Physicians who usually care for elders may be in the best position to provide short-term guidance and effective intervention. The patient is often familiar with this person and more likely to be receptive to advice from him or her.

While the Fleming contribution focuses on a framework that can be utilized by primary care physicians, the Schonfeld/Dupree chapter develops a model that is more extensive for those patients with more developed problems. They document their wealth of experience with the

Gerontology Alcohol Project (GAP) and other programs. For example, GAP treatment involves a three-phase approach. In the first phase, each patient is assessed. In the second stage, patients enter the first model of the program where they are taught to break down the various components of their drinking behavior. They learn to identify the antecedents of their own drinking behavior as well as strategies to reverse their negative behaviors and, lastly, program participants enter the final phase of treatment where they learn to master techniques of management of their behaviors. Once these stages have been completed, they may enter a 12-month follow-up program. The follow-up may consist of visits and/or telephone contact with the program participants.

Other models based on the Gerontology Alcohol Project (GAP) emerged at the Florida Mental Health Institute. A variation of the GAP program was implemented in a program for veterans in Los Angeles. The California-based program was called "GET SMART." The Schonfeld/Dupree chapter also includes case examples that illustrate their treatment models.

While the Fleming and Schonfled/Dupree chapters relate to specific program initiatives at their respective universities, Atkinson provides us with a comprehensive discussion of available treatment strategies for aging alcoholics. His contribution covers a discussion of intervention, outreach approaches, and case management. He presents successfully an inventory of various services and approaches for aging alcoholics and stresses various themes such as the importance of supportive, nonjudgmental staff attitudes and the need to treat aging problem drinkers in the total context that is cognizant of the full range of their health and social circumstances.

Dr. Atkinson also includes a helpful summary table of the various roles for the case manager in the various stages of treatment including the following: decision for abstinence and treatment, early remission, drinking relapses, and aftercare.

The concluding chapter in this part elaborates on the treatment strategies available for prescription drug misuse. At the beginning of this introduction we noted that elderly alcohol and drug misuse were distinctive categories that should be analyzed separately.

Finlayson and Hofmann describe the dimensions of psychoactive substance use within the context of addictive disorders. They state that elderly persons are at risk for prescription drug dependence as a result of medical and psychiatric comorbidity. This area of study is newer than that of alcohol misuse and is a welcome addition to this text. Different generations of elders will continue to develop varying patterns of addictive cultures for alcohol, drugs, and medications.

Therefore, in the final part of this volume, we have included chapters dealing with addiction to tobacco and gambling.

Other Addictive Disorders

The inclusion of the contribution by Boyd and Orleans is very welcome. We are all cognizant of the health consequences of excessive tobacco use. The authors outline strategies used to assist smokers in overcoming their addiction to nicotine. One notes immediately the similarity between these treatment strategies and those related to alcohol and other drugs. Health care professionals who treat elderly alcoholics often comment on the related problems in treating patients also trying to curtail nicotine addiction. The authors also note that nicotine addiction often limits the effectiveness of other medications they are taking.

The same analogy can be applied to gambling addiction. The chapter prepared by Pavalko identifies the basic characteristics of problem gambling. For example, he states that gamblers have an intense preoccupation with gambling to the point that it dominates their lives. Similar to addiction to substances, gamblers develop tolerance and may exhibit withdrawal symptoms when they try to cut back or stop gambling.

Dr. Pavalko also includes a riveting discussion about cross addiction. He notes that about half of gambling anonymous members in treatment report a serious chemical addiction (usually alcohol) at some point in their lives and for a long period of time. For example, about 20% of people receiving inpatient treatment for chemical dependency are problem gamblers. Compared with patients who did not have a gambling problem, problem gamblers are more likely to abuse alcohol, smoke cigarettes, and use marijuana. Hence, we note again, the interdependence of these addictive behaviors. The etiology, however, of cross addiction still remains undeveloped, particularly for elderly populations. Research and treatment approaches need to be developed for these groups. For this reason we are very pleased with the inclusion of these latter two chapters.

The final contribution by Coogle and Osgood calls attention to the great need for prevention programs for elder use of alcohol and substance misuse. In an earlier chapter, Dr. Fleming also called our attention to an expanding public health paradigm. Dr. Coogle and Dr. Osgood provide an excellent overview of the current thinking about substance misuse as a public health concern. Today, they state, the public health approach places greater priority on health promotion and emphasizes health education and environmental support. But to date, very few programs have focused on the primary prevention of alcoholism in older people. The statewide program in Virginia described in this chapter outlines a model which hopefully may be applied throughout the country. The aim of the project was to prevent alcohol abuse among older adults through the provision of information and education to older people, caregivers of older adults, and service providers of older adult clientele. The authors also provide us with invaluable information about the organization, management, and evaluation of such a prevention program.

We are confident that the readings contained in this text will provide invaluable guidance to health and social service personnel who deal with older people who misuse alcohol, drugs, prescription medications, and other substances. And we are hopeful that these very fine contributions by such well-known scholars and practitioners will stimulate new research and the development of other treatment models.

PART I

Recognition, Assessment, and Complications of Elderly Alcohol/Drug Misuse

2

Recognition and Assessment of Alcohol and Drug Dependence in the Elderly

David W. Oslin and Rita Holden

Introduction

There would appear to be a consensus that alcohol and drug *dependence* are disorders that justify recognition and treatment. However, there is no consensus regarding the recognition and treatment of patterns of substance use or substance use problems that *do not lead* to a diagnosis of dependence. In terms of recognition and treatment of alcohol problems, the critical first step is defining the target symptoms or target behaviors that should be identified for treatment.

Among older adults, this is an important issue because there is concern that the diagnostic criteria for alcohol and benzodiazepine dependence are difficult to apply to older adults, especially older women. For instance, older women often drink alone at home, and thus, this pattern of drinking would not lead to legal difficulties, arguments with others, or dysfunction in the workplace. Similarly, the older adult who is physiologically dependent upon a benzodiazepine and has chronic insomnia may not exhibit other symptoms of dependence. However, there is emerging evidence that these patterns of drinking or drug use for older adults are associated with physical and mental health problems. This diagnostic dilemma has led to the coining of several terms for other categories of older drinkers including "at risk drinking," "problem drinking," "heavy drinking," "medication misuse," and "abusive drinking."

While each of these terms is definable and has merit, the use of multiple diagnostic terms can lead to confusion as to how and whom to screen and what problems or patterns of use to recognize and treat. This dilemma is consistent with the studies that have demonstrated lower rates of detection and treatment of alcohol problems among older adults compared with younger adults (Curtis et al., 1986). Confusion about who does have an illness or who would benefit from an intervention not only affects physician behavior in terms of offering treatment, but also affects patients' behavior with regards to seeking treatment or acceptance of treatment recommendations. The stereotyped older patient in need of addiction treatment is the person who has drunk heavily all of his or her life, has failing health related to the alcohol, and has no social network. In contrast, the relatively healthy 70-year-old person who is drinking moderately, but has some mild cognitive loss or is struggling with blood pressure control does not think he or she is in need of help with drinking and rarely asks for assistance. This diagnostic confusion is highlighted in the following case example.

> Mr. Jones is a 72-year-old man seen by his primary care practitioner (PCP) for a routine exam. He reports suffering from some ill-described upper abdominal discomfort, but otherwise has no complaints. He currently lives by himself, does his own housework and shopping, and has a limited circle of friends. He has family, but none that live near him and he is financially able to make ends meet. Upon asking about general health habits, the PCP learns that Mr. Jones does not smoke but does drink each day at dinner and bedtime. The PCP asks him the CAGE questions, which seem to upset him, but he responds negatively to each question. His PCP makes a comment to be watchful of his drinking, but does not pursue this further. He attributes the abdominal pain to gastritis and prescribes a histamine antagonist.
>
> Six months later, at the urging of his family, the patient undergoes a mental health evaluation. The family is concerned about his ability to live alone and is considering urging him to move into an assisted living situation. During his evaluation, it is learned that he is quite functional in ability to perform daily activities, although he is somewhat slowed and rarely travels outside of the house. Cognitively, he shows no signs of dementia, but has some diminution in reaction time and problem solving. Upon questioning him about his alcohol use, it is determined that he routinely drinks one standard drink for dinner and two standard drinks of sherry before bed. This has been his pattern of drinking for 15 years since becoming a widower.

This case illustrates several of the dilemmas facing clinicians when evaluating older drinkers. Mr. Jones does not appear to have any symptoms of alcohol dependence. It is likely that his alcohol use is contributing to his gastritis, but neither the patient, PCP, nor psychiatrist made that association. Clearly he is drinking over the limits recommended by NIAAA (1 drink/day for older adults) and this would define him as an at-risk drinker. As in this case, many providers are unclear about what to recommend or how to proceed with treatment, having determined that the patient is drinking more than he should, but does not appear to be an "alcoholic."

When health care providers screen or examine a patient for an illness or a behavior, there is generally an underlying assumption that the problem for which one is screening is amenable to an intervention that will either lead to prevention of further complications, or treatment for the problem at hand. It is not unreasonable to speculate that the lack of understanding of the benefits of reduced substance use when dependence is not present, and the general belief that there are few accessible and effective treatments for substance abuse, will also significantly lower a clinician's interest in screening or recognizing problem drinking. Toward this end, there needs to be better dissemination of information regarding currently available, efficacious treatments for at-risk alcohol consumption, alcoholism and other drug abuse, as well as continued development of more effective treatments.

Moreover, for screening and recognition to be useful, everyone involved in screening and any subsequent intervention should be in agreement about the purpose. For example, if the health care provider does not think that there are older patients who meet the diagnostic criteria for alcohol dependence or that treatment will work, then it is unlikely that the physician will seek to identify the symptoms or recommend treatment even based upon a positive examination. Likewise, if the patient does not have confidence in the diagnosis or the recommendations, it is unlikely that the patient will be adherent with the recommendations. Finally, among the elderly, the diagnosis of alcohol dependence is relatively uncommon, with a prevalence of less than 4% of the general population and even less among women (Liberto, Oslin, & Ruskin, 1992). However, upwards of 10–20 percent of older adults are drinking above the recommended guidelines of no more than seven standard drinks per week and no episodes of binge drinking (four or more drinks per drinking occasion). Thus, there is potentially a large proportion of older drinkers who are "at risk" for developing problems from their alcohol consumption or who may be having isolated or focal alcohol-related problems that do not meet diagnostic criteria for dependence. The number of older adults using illicit drugs such as marijuana, cocaine, or opioids is estimated at less than 1 percent. Thus, for late-life addictions, it is not clear that mass screening for a disorder that is as rare as drug dependence, and arguably alcohol dependence and misuse of prescription and over-the-counter medications, is worth the cost both in regards to finances and time. Moreover, clinicians are likely to be lax at conducting the screening if only an occasional patient is identified.

Thus, the accurate recognition of problem behaviors and illness require that three general principles be met—(a) there is a well-defined target symptom or behavior; (b) changing the target symptoms or behavior will lead to improved health or quality of life; and (c) the target symptoms or problem are not rare events. The purpose of this chapter will be to review various targets for prevention and intervention and then review methods and instruments that will improve the recognition of these targets.

Defining the Target: What Problems Should Be Detected

At-Risk Use

At-risk substance use is defined as consumption above a specified level that may or may not meet criteria for abuse or dependence. The purpose of defining a group of individuals who meet this definition of a target pattern of use is the ability to identify a population that is at high risk of developing problems related to the alcohol or medication use, and thus do intervene in a preventive manner. This concept generally refers to alcohol or benzodiazepine use and not illicit drug use. The reason for this is that it is presumed to be rare for a person to use illicit drugs without being dependent upon them. While this may or may not be true, it is true that illicit drug use is rare among older adults, and therefore, the issue of at-risk illicit drug use is not currently germane to the elderly. The only possible exception to this is the use of marijuana. However, there are very limited estimates of the prevalence of marijuana use among the elderly, and therefore this will not be covered in this section.

At-Risk Alcohol Use

Several different organizations including the U.S. Department of Agriculture and the U.S. Department of Health and Human Services have published recommendations regarding the consumption of alcohol (U.S. Department of Agriculture/U.S. Department of Health and Human Services, 1990). The recommended safe level of alcohol consumption for healthy older adults is no more than seven standard drinks per week. A panel of experts assembled by the Center for Substance Abuse Treatment further recommended that older adults should not binge drink (CSAT, 1998). Binge drinking is generally defined as any drinking episode that includes four or more standard drinks (in younger adults the limit is usually five or more standard drinks). The consensus panel also recommends abstinence for certain individuals, including people who plan to drive or engage in other activities that require attention or skill; people taking medication, including over-the-counter medications; recovering alcoholics; and people with certain medical or psychiatric conditions such as hypertension, peptic ulcer, or depression (CSAT, 1998). An alternative target for recognition and potential treatment is to identify only those individuals who are heavy consumers of alcohol. Among the elderly, the definition of heavy use is often more than 14 to 21 standard drinks per week or more than two binge episodes per month (see Fleming's chapter for further discussion of at-risk drinking).

The rationale for such recommendations comes from mounting evidence of the risks of drinking above these recommendations (Oslin, 2000). Moderate alcohol consumption has been demonstrated to increase the risk of having a stroke caused by bleeding, although it decreases the risk of strokes caused by blocked blood vessels. Moderate alcohol use has also been demonstrated to impair driving-related skills even at low levels of consumption and it may lead to other injuries such as falls. Of particular importance to the elderly is the potential interaction between alcohol and both prescribed and over-the-counter medications, especially psychoactive medications such as benzodiazepines, barbiturates and antidepressants (see also Adam's chapter). Alcohol is also known to interfere with metabolism of medications such as digoxin and warfarin. The risk of breast cancer has been shown to increase by approximately 50% in women who consumed three to nine drinks per week compared with women who drank fewer than three drinks per week.

Of special interest to mental health providers are the effects of moderate alcohol consumption on other mental health disorders. In a recent study of over 2000 elderly patients, Oslin and colleagues demonstrated an added benefit of reduction in moderate alcohol use during treatment of a depressive disorder (Oslin, Katz, Edell, & TenHave, 2000). This study defined moderate alcohol use as one to seven drinks per week. The study further demonstrated that the greater the alcohol consumption, the larger the effect on the treatment of depression. Although data are lacking, there is speculation that moderate alcohol use may have a negative effect on the prognosis, and course, of dementing illnesses such as Alzheimer's Disease. Moreover, alcohol use may exacerbate or lead to personality changes or behavioral disturbances in patients with dementia.

Confounding the use of moderate drinking levels as targets for treatment is the potential benefit of moderate alcohol consumption, especially with regard to cardiovascular disease (Rimm et al., 1991; Stampfer, Colditz, Willett, Speizer, & Hennekens, 1988; Thun et al., 1997). Alcohol in moderate amounts may improve self-esteem or provide relaxation. Alcohol is often consumed socially and may help to reduce stress (Dufour, Archer, & Gordis, 1992). A more recent study of drinking practices among community dwelling older adults found that the greater the number of drinks consumed per day, the higher their scores on a depression scale (Graham & Schmidt, 1999). The frequency of drinking was not related to depression, suggesting that binge drinking was a more significant factor. There is growing evidence that among otherwise healthy adults, especially middle-aged adults, moderate alcohol use may reduce disability associated with cardiovascular disease and reduce the risk of developing a dementing illness (Broe et al., 1998; Rimm et al., 1991). Thus, in the absence of alcohol dependence, clinicians may feel confused as to whether they should recommend to their moderate drinking patients either no change in consumption or a reduction in consumption. In support of this concept, Conigliaro and colleagues surveyed patients of all age groups identified as "problem drinkers" who recently had a primary care visit (Conigliaro, Lofgren, & Hanusa, 1998). The majority of the patients remembered having a discussion with their doctor about drinking, but only half remembered being advised to reduce their drinking.

At-Risk Benzodiazepine or Other Prescription Medication Use

Benzodiazepine and other prescription medications pose a different problem in terms of defining at risk use. Pharmaceutical data clearly show that benzodiazepines are prescribed more often to elderly patients and that the older a patient is, the more likely he or she is to be receiving multiple medications (Golden et al., 1999; Lasslia et al., 1996). Indeed the average elderly patient is taking 5.3 prescription medications each day (Golden et al., 1999). Stoehr and colleagues also have found that 87 percent of the elderly report regular use of over-the-counter medications and 5.7 percent are taking five or more over-the-counter medications (Stoehr, Ganguli, Seaberg, Echement, & Belle, 1997). These figures are also likely to be underestimates, as they typically do not include herbal remedy use. The difficulty with defining at-risk use for medications is determining what is *appropriate* use. As clinicians, each time we prescribe or recommend a treatment there are certain risks and benefits to that treatment. Properly weighed, this ratio should favor a benefit.

Having said this, certain medications are associated with greater risk than others. For instance, benzodiazepines have been demonstrated to increase the risk of falls and thus fractures; they can cause impairment to driving skills, disrupt sleep cycles, and, among the frail elderly, cause excessive disability (Hemmelgarn, Suissa, Huang, Boivin, & Pinard, 1997; Herings, Stricker, deBoer, Bakker, & Sturmans, 1995; Newman, Enright, Manolio, Haponik, & Whal, 1997). Similarly, the antihistamine diphenhydramine has been shown to produce cognitive deficits in healthy elderly, raising the possibility of inducing excessive cognitive deficits when prescribed in patients with dementing illnesses (Katz et al., 1998). The exposure to these risks is heightened when the medication is used for a longer duration than intended or warranted, or when the medication is improperly prescribed by giving an excessive dose or having been prescribed for the wrong indication. Examples among the elderly include prolonged use of sedative medications such as benzodiazepines or diphenhydramine for insomnia, use of antianxiety medications for the treatment of depression or chronic pain, and the use of high doses of antipsychotics for the treatment of behavioral disturbances associated with dementia. The following case history exemplifies the difficulty in determining problem medication use:

> Ms. Smith is a 76-year-old African American female who recently signed on with an HMO medicare plan that required her to see a new PCP. On her initial visit with her new PCP, her medications were reviewed and she was noted to be taking a benzodiazepine (temazepam, 15 mg) each night for insomnia as well as a variety of other medications. Ms. Smith said that she

had been taking the temazepam for several years and that it helps to relax her. She denied being depressed or having lost interest in activities. She reports that her energy is good and that she sleeps throughout the night except to urinate. She has never tried to go to sleep without her medication because she knows the importance of taking her medication as prescribed. There are no notes from her previous physician that indicate a beneficial response to the benzodiazepine or the purpose of the original prescription. Her medical problems include chronic obstructive lung disease, arthritis for which she uses a cane, and well-controlled hypertension.

This patient would not meet criteria for benzodiazepine dependence but is being exposed to the risks of prolonged use. She also is likely to have developed physical dependence on the medication and would have the potential to exhibit withdrawal symptoms upon abrupt discontinuation. The new physician was appropriately concerned about the long-term use of this medication. He also appropriately inquired about possible depression. The patient does have both a respiratory disorder and a gait disturbance that can be affected by her long-term benzodiazepine use, but again it is not clear that the physician recognized these as issues for this patient. Nor is it clear whether any attempt was made to decrease or discontinue her temazepam. Thus, at-risk medication use is not best described as a threshold of consumption that should be avoided, but rather as a threshold of consumption that warrants an evaluation of the medical necessity of the medication. Conceptually, a threshold can be set for both dose and duration of exposure. This would allow detection of patients who are taking high doses of medication and also are on medications longer than would be reasonable clinical practice. For benzodiazepines, barbiturates and opioids, a recommendation to address patterns of near daily use that lasts for more than 3 months in elderly patients was made as part of a multisite collaborative project funded by the Substance Abuse and Mental Health Services Administration and the Department of Veterans Affairs. This recommendation was made based upon expert opinion and would need validation as a target definition for at-risk use. Other medications such as antidepressants, H2 blockers or nonsteroidal medications may require different definitions for targeting at-risk use.

Problem Use

Problem use is broadly defined as the consumption of alcohol or the use of medications or drugs that has already led to at least one definable problem or adverse consequence. The identified problem(s) may or may not be sufficient to warrant a diagnosis of substance dependence. However, these problems are often sufficient to meet criteria for a DSM–IV diagnosis of substance abuse but not dependence (see Table 2.1). One of the rationales for using this definition for a target of intervention is the ease in operationalizing the definition. To meet these criteria, there is some level of consumption of the drug, alcohol, or medication and the

Table 2.1 DSM–IV Criteria for Substance Abuse and Dependence (American Psychiatric Association, 1994)

Abuse

A. A maladaptive pattern of substance use leading to clinically significant impairment or distress, as manifested by one or more of the following, occurring within a 12-month period:
    1. Failure to fulfill major social, educational, or occupational roles
    2. Recurrent use in situations that are physically hazardous
    3. Recurrent substance-related legal problems
    4. Continued use despite having persistent or recurrent social or interpersonal problems caused or exacerbated by the effects of the substance.

B. The symptoms have never met the criteria for Substance Dependence for this class of substance.

Dependence

A maladaptive pattern of substance use leading to clinically significant impairment or distress, as manifested by three (or more) of the following, occurring at any time in the same 12-month period:

1. Tolerance as defined by either of the following:
    a. a need for markedly increased amounts of the substance to achieve intoxication or the desired effect
    b. markedly diminished effect with continued use of the same amount of the substance
2. Withdrawal, as manifested by either of the following:
    a. the characteristic withdrawal syndrome for the substance
    b. the same (or a closely relataed) substance is taken to relieve or avoid withdrawal symptoms
3. Substance is often taken in larger amounts or over a longer period of time than was intended
4. Persistent desire or attempts to cut down or control substance use
5. Great deal of time spent in activities necessary to obtain the substance or recover from its effects
6. Important social, occupational, or recreational activities are given up or reduced because of substance use
7. Continued use despite adverse health consequences.

patient has at least one problem that generally comes from a standardized list. For example, any alcohol use complicating diabetes mellitus, hypertension, or depression, or leading to an arrest for drinking and driving, marital conflict, or financial problems. Of note, this method does not assume that the alcohol, medication, or drug was the sole cause of the problem but rather that there is a high likelihood that the use led to or exacerbated the problem.

Substance Dependence

The current definition of substance dependence in the Diagnostic and Statistical Manual Fourth Edition (DSM–IV) is outlined in Table 2.1 (American Psychiatric Association, 1994). The DSM–IV diagnostic criteria are based on knowledge of young to middle-age adults and have undergone minimal validation in older persons. Because of this lack of validation and concern that the symptoms offered as examples in DSM–IV do not relate to older adults, many authors feel that the DSM–IV criteria are difficult to apply and may not be valid in older populations. This may be particularly true of benzodiazepine abuse and dependence.

Irrespective of the problems with the DSM–IV criteria, several other factors must be considered when applying these criteria. The DSM–IV diagnostic criteria rely greatly upon self-reported behavioral symptoms. Self-report has the potential for bias due to memory impairments, lack of insight, or unwillingness to admit symptoms. There are several other factors that impact upon poor reliability of diagnosing substance use disorders among older patients, including: a poor understanding of the disorders by clinicians, denial on the part of the physician or the family, and a belief that treatment is ineffective and therefore diagnosing the disorder is futile. When utilizing the diagnostic criteria, collateral information from other sources such as family, friends, or employers, is an important source of clinical information either to challenge or confirm what the patient reports. Further validation of DSM–IV diagnostic criteria for substance use disorders in older patients is necessary. Research on the use of collateral sources of information, the use of quantity and frequency of substance use, and the use of clinical signs to improve the validity and reliability of DSM–IV diagnostic criteria among older patients is also justified.

Assessment and Recognition

Having defined the target symptoms, behaviors or problems that one wishes to recognize, it is important to determine how to recognize the symptoms or syndrome. To reiterate an earlier observation, we recognize only what we seek to recognize and thus asking the patient about his or her alcohol or drug use and medication use is an imperative first step. That said, the quantity and frequency of use of alcohol or drugs is only as good as the self-report. Thus, the validity of the self-reported information must be accounted for in any clinical decision. Self-report may underestimate alcohol or drug use, given that denial plays a role in the pathology of alcoholism and people's ability to remember past events or report past average consumption may deteriorate with age and with long-standing use or abuse of alcohol or drugs. Despite these problems, Werch's study of an elder age group found that retrospective self-report was as reliable as a prospective diet record in identifying patterns of alcohol use (Werch, 1989).

Assessment of the quantity and frequency of alcohol or drug use has been conducted in three basic ways: questions regarding average consumption practices, retrospective reporting of use on a day-by-day basis for some defined period of time (the time-line follow-back method (TLFB), and prospective monitoring and recording of alcohol and drug use. Only one article in the literature examines the reliability and validity of these methods in the elderly although there are several such articles dealing with younger patients (Werch, 1989). The prospective diary method has been shown to record the greatest amount of consumption and in younger adults is closest to matching sales data for alcohol beverages (Lemmens, Tan, & Knibbe, 1992). Thus, the prospective diary is considered the "gold standard." However, this method is impractical for screening or brief assessments as it would require multiple visits and is rather time consuming in terms of explaining the diary, collecting the diaries, etc.

The TLFB method is used the most in research studies of treatment for addiction and has become the standard for such studies (Sobell & Sobell, 1992). Among older adults a 7-day TLFB method has been shown to correlate well with the prospective diary. However, two difficulties arise in using this method. First, there is a possibility that the week of measurement is not representative of the persons' "usual" drinking. The second problem relates to low frequency users. For nondrinkers or nearly-every-day drinkers, the TLFB closely matches the prospective diary method (Lemmens et al., 1992). At less frequent use the TLFB slightly underestimates use. It also takes longer to administer than average frequency and is not particularly amenable to self-assessment. Interviewer-administered questions are felt to be more accurate with regards to determining standard drink equivalents, because patients can self-define "one drink" as anything from a one ounce shot to an 8-ounce glass of liquor. General questions about the average quantity and frequency of use are least likely to match prospective diary consumption reports and are felt to underestimate moderate drinking.

Assessing quantity and frequency of use has the advantage of ease of administration. Therefore, it is not surprising that most clinicians appraise the severity of alcohol use by measuring thc quantity and frequency of alcohol consumed over a defined time period. Quantity and frequency of use can be used independently to screen and identify patients defined as at-risk. However, quantity and frequency must be combined with other measures when attempting to recognize problem drinking or a diagnosis of substance abuse or dependence. This is because quantity and frequency of drinking are inadequate in identifying how alcohol is affecting a patient psychologically, socially, or physiologically. Indeed, among older drinkers, moderate consumption has been demonstrated to be a particularly poor indicator of the presence or absence of a diagnosis of alcohol abuse or dependence (Grant & Harford, 1989).

Standardized Screening Instruments

Although the informal interview remains the clinician's greatest asset, self-administered questionnaires provide the busy clinician with a rapid, sensitive, and low-cost method of screening for problem use, aiding the clinician to concentrate attention on the patients most likely to suffer from the target symptoms or disorder of interest. Several measures of alcohol-related problems exist and some have been examined in the elderly. Self-assessment methods include the CAGE,[1] the Alcohol Use

1. C-Have you ever tried to ***Cut*** down on your drinking? A-Have you gotten *Annoyed* at someone telling you about your drinking? G-Do you feel ***Guilty*** about your drinking? E-Do you need an ***Eyeopener*** (drink in the morning)?

Disorders Identification Test (AUDIT), the Michigan Alcohol Screening Test—Geriatric Version (GMAST), and the Michigan Alcohol Screening Test (MAST). Structured interview-based assessment methods include the Diagnostic Interview Schedule (DIS), Structured Clinical Interview for DSM–IV (SCID-IV), and Semi-Structured Assessment of the Genetics of Alcoholism (SSAGA) (for a review, see CSAT, 1998). The interview-based assessments are generally lengthy and possibly underestimate diagnosis in the elderly because of the aforementioned problems with relevance of some diagnostic criteria to age group. The self-assessment instruments have been validated in the elderly. Buchsbaum and colleagues found that a score of one or greater on the CAGE questionnaire had a sensitivity of 86 percent and a specificity of 78 percent in elderly medical outpatients (Buchsbaum, Buchanan, Welsh, Centor, & Schnoll, 1992). Similarly, Jones and colleagues found an 88 percent sensitivity and specificity for a CAGE score of one in elderly medical outpatients (Jones, Lindsey, Yount, Soltys, & Farani-enayat, 1993). The MAST and AUDIT have lower sensitivity and specificity (Buchsbaum et al., 1992; Jones et al., 1993; Moran, Naughton, & Hughes, 1990; Saunders, AAsland, Babor, Delafuente, & Grant, 1993). Most recently, Blow and colleagues developed a geriatric version of the MAST, a short form of which is presented in Table 2.2, and in preliminary data have found a 95 percent sensitivity and 78 percent specificity for identifying older alcoholics (Blow, 1993). Widespread clinical use of the GMAST has not occurred and the short form will need further validation. However, given its focus on issues related to aging and potential usefulness of the instrument for treatment planning, it would have to be the primary recommendation. Instruments that use information from families and friends also need to be developed.

Biological markers of alcohol use have proved to be less accepted in clinical practice but can be useful. There are several laboratory values that indicate recent use or abuse such as a blood alcohol level or an acetate level, which is a metabolite of alcohol (Salaspuro, 1994). Long-term markers of disease include the following: gamma-glutamyl transferase (GGT), a liver function measure which has a low sensitivity and a moderate specificity for diagnosing an alcohol use disorder, a measure of red blood cell size, the mean corpuscular volume, which has a low sensitivity but a high specificity; high density lipoprotein (HDL) level, a component of blood cholesterol, which shows a linear increase with alcohol use; and carbohydrate-deficient transferrin (CDT) which has a moderate sensitivity and moderate specificity (Oslin et al., 1998). For

Table 2.2 Short Michigan Alcohol Screening Test—Geriatric Version (SMAST-G)

In the past year:	YES	NO
1. When talking with others, do you ever underestimate how much you actually drink?	___ (1)	___ (0)
2. After a few drinks, have you sometimes not eaten or been able to skip a meal because you didn't feel hungry?	___ (1)	___ (0)
3. Does having a few drinks help decrease your shakiness or tremors?	___ (1)	___ (0)
4. Does alcohol sometimes make it hard for you to remember parts of the day or night?	___ (1)	___ (0)
In the past year:		
5. Do you usually take a drink to relax or calm your nerves?	___ (1)	___ (0)
6. Do you drink to take your mind off your problems?	___ (1)	___ (0)
7. Have you ever increased your drinking after experiencing a loss in your life?	___ (1)	___ (0)
8. Has a doctor or nurse ever said they were worried or concerned about your drinking?	___ (1)	___ (0)
9. Have you ever made rules to manage your drinking?	___ (1)	___ (0)
10. When you feel lonely, does having a drink help?	___ (1)	___ (0)
TOTAL SMAST-G SCORE (0–10)		_____

Three or more positive responses are indicative of an alcohol use problem.

Note. From "The Michigan Alcoholism Screening Test—Geriatric Version (MAST–G): A New Elderly-Specific Screening Instrument," by F. C. Blow, K. J. Brower, J. E. Schulenberg, L. M. Demo-Dananberg, J. P. Young, and T. P. Beresford, 1992, *Alcoholism: Clinical and Experimental Research, 16*(2), p. 372. Reprinted with permission of the University of Michigan Alcohol Research Center.

medications and drugs of abuse, urine drug screens continue to be useful as both a screening tool and as a confirmation of self-report. The majority of drugs of abuse will remain detectable in a urine drug screen for 4 or more days and some for several weeks.

Other unproven clinical markers suggestive of substance abuse in the elderly rely on identification of related medical or psychiatric disorders as an indicator of disease. As an example, a patient who presents for a dementia evaluation with a history of malnutrition and a vitamin B12 deficiency anemia should alert a clinician to the possibility of an alcohol use disorder, because such disorders are often associated with these other findings. Psychosocial signs such as legal and family difficulties, loss of employment, persistent depression, or social isolation are also potentially useful indicators but do not negate the need to question patients about drug and alcohol use.

Detailed Clinical Evaluation

Once patients have been recognized as having significant drinking problems or have been identified as being at-risk for drinking problems, a more detailed and comprehensive addiction-focused evaluation is warranted. This comprehensive evaluation should focus on all aspects of the patient's life including social and environmental strengths and stressors and physical and mental functioning. While the content of this exam is similar to a good clinical evaluation, special attention should be paid to problems known to be caused by alcohol use. This includes gathering sufficient information to diagnose alcohol abuse or dependence. In general, heavy drinking and alcohol dependence can lead to a wide variety of physical health problems including liver disease, alcohol-related dementia, and cardiomyopathy. Heavy drinking and alcohol dependence can also exacerbate a number of physical health disorders such as cerebrovascular accidents (strokes), chronic obstructive lung disease, hypertension, and diabetes.

The physical examination for a patient who is a significant drinker would include a focused neurologic exam evoking evidence of peripheral neuropathy, cranial nerve dysfunction, and a cognitive assessment. The clinician should also focus the examination on the liver, spleen, cardiovascular system, and any evidence of trauma that may have occurred from falls, and so on. In addition to recording blood pressure (for hypertension) and weight (for evidence of malnutrition), the following laboratory studies are recommended during an initial examination or annual follow-up examination.

1. Complete blood count—macrocytic anemia is often associated with heavy drinking.
2. Liver studies (AST, ALT, and GGT)—elevations in any of these tests may be indicative of liver fibrosis or early liver failure. In patients who have abnormal elevations in these tests, especially GGT, the lab value can be used to track progress in treatment.
3. Albumin—is a marker of malnutrition and can be a sign of severe alcoholism.

Since persons who are heavy drinkers are more likely to also have poor nutritional habits, it is common to recommend to these patients the addition of a multivitamin to their diet. Thiamine deficiency is a particular concern for heavy drinkers because this deficiency can lead to the neurologic disorder known as Wernicke-Korsakoff syndrome. This syndrome has the principal features of dementia and psychotic symptoms. Therefore, it is also recommended that heavy drinkers be started on thiamine supplementation. Vitamins and thiamine in particular can be recommended for longer periods of time when patients continue to drink or when there is evidence of malnutrition or cognitive impairment.

A thorough mental status examination should also be included in a comprehensive examination. The interactions between alcohol use and depression and anxiety are complex. Alcohol use can cause depression and anxiety as well as be a reaction to the presence of depression or anxiety. Key steps include assessing the level of distress present and deciding what steps should be taken to address patient distress. Measuring symptoms of anxiety or depression can be done with any of a number of standardized instruments including the Hamilton Rating Scale for Depression, the Hamilton Rating Scale for Anxiety, the Center for Epidemiologic Studies—Depression Scale, the Beck Depression Inventory, or General Health Questionnaire (Goldberg, 1978; Hamilton, 1960; Radloff, 1977; Beck & Steer, 1987). In treating patients for alcohol problems, be careful not to ignore symptoms that do not meet diagnostic criteria as these depressive or anxious symptoms can have significant impact on treatment outcomes for drinking. Of particular concern here is the combination of suicidal ideation and either depression or drinking. Both depression and drinking are strongly associated with completed suicide, especially in the elderly. The presence of moderate or severe depression or heavy drinking should always be followed by questions regarding suicide risk. A key in treating patients with these more complex presentations or symptoms is to recognize your own limitations for providing care and to seek assistance through consultation or referral.

Discussion

As previously discussed, one of the cornerstones to recognition of a behavior or disease is the belief by the clinician that he or she can recommend an effective intervention. Once identified, many clinicians feel ill-equipped to treat alcoholism, especially in older adults. Studies have shown that for adults of all ages, 11 percent to 96 percent of patients referred for addiction treatment actually called or started treatment (Wiseman, Henderson, & Briggs, 1997). The rate for older adults is unknown but can be inferred to be low as there are few older adults in treatment programs compared to the number with alcoholism. Although there tends to be a general belief that addiction treatment is futile or of limited benefit and that addiction treatment needs to occur in highly specialized settings, recent evidence suggests otherwise. Among patients with alcohol dependence, there has been remarkable progress made in the last decade in the development of effective pharmacological and nonpharmacological treatments (see part Two in this volume). Treatment planning does not have to be complex and starts in the primary care office. Studies have demonstrated that brief advice is an effective first step in managing uncontrolled drinking (see Fleming's chapter). Older patients often do not recognize the dangers of their alcohol consumption and simple direct advice may be all that is needed to motivate them to become abstinent.

In one of the largest nonpharmacological treatment studies ever conducted, three different short-term outpatient psychosocial treatments were found to be highly and equally effective in reducing alcohol consumption among adults with alcohol dependence (7% of whom were age 60 or over) (Project MATCH Research Group, 1997). Age was not a significant factor in determining treatment outcome. In 1995, naltrexone became the first pharmacological treatment for alcoholism approved by the FDA in over 50 years. Naltrexone has been shown in several clinical trials to be safe and efficacious in preventing relapse among alcohol-dependent patients (Oslin, Liberto, O'Brien, Krois, & Norbeck, 1997; Volpicelli, Alterman, Hayashida, & O'Brien, 1992). Naltrexone has also been studied among older adults and found to have similar efficacy (Oslin et al., 1997). Current studies are being conducted to test the effectiveness of naltrexone in primary care settings. Among moderate drinkers, recent studies by Fleming and colleagues and Barry and colleagues suggest that primary care-based physician advice is effective in reducing alcohol consumption in older adult patients (Barry et al., 1998; Fleming, Barry, Adams, & Stauffacher, 1999) (see also Fleming's chapter).

In conclusion, there is evidence for a high prevalence of older adults who are drinking at levels that are, or could in some time become, harmful to their health. Thus, screening for these individuals is justified, as there are established treatments available for reducing alcohol consumption among older adults. What appears to be needed, however, is a better understanding among clinicians and patients of the risks associated with moderate to heavy alcohol consumption, especially in the face of other chronic physical or mental health problems. Until these concepts are better understood by the community of providers, interventions will continue to be considered only for those with the most severe of problems.

Acknowledgment

Research for this chapter was supported, in part, by a grant from the National Institute of Mental Health (#) 1K08MH 01599.

References

American Psychiatric Association. (1994). *Diagnostic and statistical manual of mental disorders,* (4th ed.). Washington, DC: Author.

Barry, K. L., Blow, F. C., Walton, M. A., Chernack, S. T., Mudd, S. A., Coyne, J. C., & Gomberg, E. S. L. (1998). Elder-specific brief alcohol intervention: 3-month outcomes. *Alcoholism: Clinical and Experimental Research, 22,* 32 A.

Beck, A. T., & Steer, R. (1987). The Beck depression inventory manual. San Antonio, TX: Psychological Corporation, Harcourt Brace Jovanovich.

Blow, F. (1993). *A geriatric version of the MAST.* Paper presented at the American Association of Geriatric Psychiatry, New Orleans, LA.

Blow, F. C., Brower, K. J., Schulenberg, J. E., Demo-Dananberg, L. M., Young, J. P., & Beresford, T. P. (1992). The Michigan Alcoholism Screening Test–Geriatric Version (MAST–G): A new elderly-specific screening instrument. *Alcoholism: Clinical and Experimental Research, 16*(2), 372.

Broe, G. A., Creasey, H., Jorm, A. F., Bennett, H. P., Casey, B., Waite, L. M., & Grayson, D. (1998). Health habits and risk of cognitive impairment and dementia. *Australian & New Zealand Journal of Public Health, 22*(5), 621–623.

Buchsbaum, D. G., Buchanan, R., Welsh, J., Centor, R., & Schnoll, S. (1992). Screening for drinking disorders in the elderly using the CAGE questionnaire. *Journal of the American Geriatric Society, 40,* 662–665.

Center for Substance Abuse Treatment. (1998). *Substance abuse among older Americans* (DHHS No. SMA 98–3179). Washington, DC: U.S. Government Printing Office.

Conigliaro, J., Lofgren, R. P., & Hanusa, B. H. (1998). Screening for problem drinking: Impact on physician behavior and patient drinking habits. *Journal of General Internal Medicine, 13,* 251–256.

Curtis, J., Millman, E., Joseph, M., Charles, J., & Bajwa, W. K. (1986). Prevalence rates for alcoholism, associated depression and dementia on the Harlem hospital medicine and surgery services. *Advances in Alcohol and Substance Abuse, 6,* 45–65.

Dufour, M. C., Archer, L., & Gordis, E. (1992). Alcohol and the elderly. *Clinics in Geriatric Medicine, 8,* 127–141.

Fleming, M. F., Barry, K. L., Adams, W. L., & Stauffacher, E. A. (1999). Brief physician advice for alcohol problems in older adults: a randomized community-based trial. *Journal of Family Practice, 48,* 378–384.

Golden, A. G., Preston, R. A., Barnett, S. D., Llorente, M., Hamdan, K., & Silverman, M. A. (1999). Inappropriate medication prescribing in homebound older adults. *Journal of the American Geriatrics Society, 47,* 948–953.

Goldberg, D. (1978). *Manual of the general health questionnaire.* Windsor, England: National Foundation for Educational Research.

Graham, K., & Schmidt, G. (1999). Alcohol use and psychosocial well-being among older adults. *Journal of Studies on Alcohol, 60,* 345–351.

Grant, B. F., & Harford, T. C. (1989). The relationship between ethanol intake and DSM-III alcohol use disorders: A cross-perspective analysis. *Journal of Substance Abuse, 1,* 231–252.

Hamilton, M. (1960). "A rating scale for depression." *Journal of Neurology, Neurosurgery, and Psychiatry, 23,* 56–65.

Hemmelgarn, B., Suissa, S., Huang, A., Boivin, J. F., & Pinard, G. (1997). Benzodiazepine use and the risk of motor vehicle crash in the elderly [see comments]. *Journal of the American Medical Association, 278*(1), 27–31.

Herings, R. M. C., Stricker, B. H. C., deBoer, A., Bakker, A., & Sturmans, F. (1995). Benzodiazepines and the risk of falling leading to femur fractures. *Archives of Internal Medicine, 155,* 1801–1807.

Jones, T. V., Lindsey, B. A., Yount, P., Soltys, R., & Farani-Enayat, B. (1993). Alcoholism screening questions: Are they valid in elderly medical outpatients. *Journal of General Internal Medicine, 8,* 674–678.

Katz, I. R., Sands, L. P., Bilker, W., DiFilippo, S., Boyce, A., & D'Angelo, K. (1998). Identification of medications that cause cognitive impairment in older people: The role of oxybutynin chloride. *Journal of the American Geriatrics Society, 46,* 8–13.

Lasslia, H. C., Stoehr, G. P., Ganguli, M., Seaberg, E. C., Gilby, J. E., Belle,

S. H., & Echement, D. A. (1996). Use of prescription medications in an elderly rural population: The MoVIES project. *Annals of Pharmacotherapy, 30,* 589–595.

Lemmens, P., Tan, E. S., & Knibbe, R. A. (1992). Measuring quantity and frequency of drinking in a general population survey: a comparison of five indices. *Journal of Studies on Alcohol, 53*(5), 476–86.

Liberto, J. G., Oslin, D. W., & Ruskin, P. E. (1992). Alcoholism in older persons: A review of the literature. *Hospital & Community Psychiatry, 43*(10), 975–84.

Moran, M. B., Naughton, B. J., & Hughes, S. (1990). Screening elderly veterans for alcoholism. *Journal of General Internal Medicine, 5,* 361–364.

Newman, A., Enright, P., Manolio, T., Haponik, E., & Whal, P. (1997). Sleep disturbances, psychosocial correlates, and cardiovascular disease in 5201 older adults: The cardiovasular health study. *Journal of the American Geriatrics Society, 45,* 1–7.

Oslin, D. (2000). Alcohol use in late life—disability and comorbity. *Journal of Geriatric Psychiatry and Neurology, 13*(3), 134–140.

Oslin, D., Katz, I., Edell, W., & TenHave, T. (2000). The effects of alcohol consumption on the treatment of depression among the elderly. *American Journal of Geriatric Psychiatry, 8,* 215–220.

Oslin, D., Liberto, J., O'Brien, J., Krois, S., & Norbeck, J. (1997). Naltrexone as an adjunctive treatment for older patients with alcohol dependence. *American Journal of Geriatric Psychiatry, 5,* 324–332.

Oslin, D. W., Pettinati, H. M., Luck, G., Semwanga, A., Cnaan, A., & O'Brien, C. P. (1998). Clinical correlations with carbohydrate-deficient transferrin levels in women with alcoholism. *Alcoholism, Clinical & Experimental Research, 22*(9), 1981–5.

Project MATCH Research Group. (1997). Matching alcoholism treatments to client heterogeneity—Project Match posttreatment drinking outcomes. *Journal of Studies on Alcohol, 58,* 7–29.

Radloff, L. (1977). "The CES-D Scale: A self-report depression scale for research in the general population." *Applied Psychological Measurement, 1,* 385–401.

Rimm, E. B., Giovannucci, E. L., Willett, W. C., Colditz, G. A., Ascherio, A., Rosner, B., & Stampfer, M. J. (1991). Prospective study of alcohol consumption and risk of coronary disease in men. *Lancet, 338,* 464–468.

Salaspuro, M. (1994). Biological state markers of alcohol abuse. *Alcohol Health and Research World, 18*(2), 131–135.

Saunders, J. B., AAsland, O. G., Babor, T. F., Delafuente, J. R., & Grant, M. (1993). Development of the alcohol-use disorders identification test (AUDIT)–WHO collaborative project on early detection of persons with harmful alcohol consumption. *Addiction, 88,* 791–804.

Sobell, L. C., & Sobell, M. B. Timeline follow-back: A technique for assessing self-reported alcohol consumption. In R. Litten, & J. Allen, *Measuring alcohol consumption* (pp. 41–65). Totowa, NJ: Humana Press, Inc.

Stampfer, M. J., Colditz, G. A., Willett, W. C., Speizer, F. E., & Hennekens, C. H. (1988). A prospective study of moderate alcohol consumption and the risk of coronary disease and stroke in women. *New England Journal of Medicine, 319,* 267–273.

Stoehr, G. P., Ganguli, M., Seaberg, E. C., Echement, D. A., & Belle, S. (1997). Over-the-counter medication use in an older rural communtity: The MoVIES project. *Journal of the American Geriatrics Society, 45,* 158–165.

Thun, M. J., Peto, R., Lopez, A. D., Monaco, J. H., Henley, S. J., Heath, C. W., & Doll, R. (1997) Alcohol consumption and mortality among middle-aged and elderly U.S. adults. *New England Journal of Medicine, 337,* 1705–1714.

U.S. Department of Agriculture/U.S. Department of Health and Human Services. (1990). *Nutrition and your health: Dietary guidelines for Americans* (3rd ed.). Washington, DC: U.S. Government Printing Office.

Volpicelli, J. R., Alterman, A. I., Hayashida, M., & O'Brien, C. P. (1992). Naltrexone in the treatment of alcohol dependence. *Archives of General Psychiatry, 49,* 876–880.

Werch, C. (1989). Quantity-frequency and diary measures of alcohol consumption for elderly drinkers. *International Journal of the Addictions, 24,* 859–865.

Wiseman, E. J., Henderson, K. L., & Briggs, M. J. (1997). Outcomes of patients in a VA ambulatory detoxification program. *Psychiatric Services, 48,* 200–203.

3

The Effects of Alcohol on Medical Illnesses and Medication Interactions

Wendy L. Adams

The Spectrum of Alcohol-Related Medical Illness

Mrs. R. was an 84-year-old woman who came to the urinary incontinence clinic because of increasing urinary urge incontinence and occasional fecal incontinence. She had been brought in by her daughter and was seated in a wheelchair. Her incontinence had worsened gradually over the past several months. During that time she had also developed a gait problem. She was unsteady on her feet, had numbness of both feet and some pain in her soles on standing. She was also sleepy a great deal of the day. She had developed swelling of both legs in the course of the last 6 months. The physical examination showed somewhat poor personal hygiene. Blood pressure was 182/94. The liver was enlarged. There was edema of both legs below the knees. She had decreased sensation in a stocking distribution below both knees. She was barely able to stand with the assistance of 2 people and was very unsteady. Her recent memory was mildly impaired and her score on the Mini Mental State Exam was 25 out of a possible 30. Laboratory testing showed a moderate anemia with a hemoglobin of 9.2 and enlarged red blood cells with a mean corpuscular volume of 108. Sodium was low at 129 and potassium was also low at 3.1. Liver function tests were moderately elevated.

As you have probably guessed, the patient described above was a heavy drinker. She was consuming 12 cans of beer each day. Interestingly, she herself had not considered that to be heavy drinking. Though her daughter suspected the alcohol consumption might be contributing to her medical problems, the patient had previously been evaluated by a general internist and a neurologist and neither had discussed alcohol use with the patient or her daughter. We advised her to discontinue alcohol use and had a home health nurse visit to monitor her for signs of withdrawal and to help manage her multiple health problems. Her daughter was also available for lengthy daily visits to monitor her functioning and assist with personal care. As she gradually regained her health, a physical therapist also worked with her to increase strength and improve balance. Fortunately, most of her symptoms improved quite dramatically within a month and she was able to continue to live independently as she strongly desired.

Alcohol may affect virtually any body system. Alcoholic liver disease is probably the most widely recognized medical complication of alcoholism, but serious damage to the nervous system, the cardiovascular system, the gastrointestinal system, bone, and muscle also occurs quite commonly. Some illnesses, such as hypertension, can result from as little as 2–3 drinks per day. Others, such as peripheral neuropathy and myopathies, probably require much higher doses of alcohol. There is a great deal of individual variation in susceptibility to the effects of alcohol, though in general women are subject to medical illness at lower amounts than men. Women are at risk of cirrhosis with consumption of 2–3 drinks per day. As the case of Mrs. R. demonstrates, alcoholics and heavy drinkers often have more than one complication simultaneously. In elderly people, alcohol-induced illness may present as "geriatric syndromes" such as incontinence, gait disturbances, and dementia. Mrs. R., for instance, had cognitive impairment, cerebellar ataxia, hypertension, fatty liver, urinary incontinence, anemia, and electrolyte disturbances that all responded to alcohol cessation. Alcohol-induced illness is often reversible, especially if it is discovered early. We need to keep heavy drinking in the differential diagnosis for many medical illnesses and geriatric syndromes and address the problem with our patients. This chapter will highlight some of the most common medical complications of heavy drinking with a special emphasis on those most important to elderly people.

Neurologic and Muscular Sequella of Heavy Drinking

> Mrs. M. was a 76-year-old woman referred for geriatric assessment because of cognitive decline. Her mental status seemed to fluctuate somewhat from visit to visit, but it was clear to her doctor that her brain function was not normal. A workup for reversible causes of dementia had been negative, including thyroid function, vitamin B12 level, electrolytes, liver and kidney function, and brain imaging. One week before her geriatric clinic appointment, Mrs. M. was stopped by the police for driving under the influence of alcohol. The police officer was immediately aware that this woman's cognition was more impaired than her intoxication accounted for and brought her to the emergency room for evaluation. Her blood alcohol level was 200 mg/dl (the legal limit for drunken driving is 80 or 100 mg/dl, varying from state to state). After detoxification she had persistent mild global cognitive deficits as well as an unstable gait due to weakness of lower extremity muscles.

Alcohol is directly toxic to nerve and muscle. In addition, the nutritional deficiencies that often accompany alcoholism can damage the nervous system and muscle. Excessive alcohol consumption may affect the brain, the autonomic nervous system or peripheral nerves. Thinking, balance, and mobility may be affected. Muscle degeneration leads to weakness and further deterioration of strength and mobility. It appears that moderately heavy drinking does not cause decline in neuromuscular functioning (Lacroix, Guralnik, Berkman, Wallace, & Satterfield, 1993; Nelson, Nevitt, Scott, Stone, & Cummings, 1994). The threshold at which damage occurs has not been established, but consumption of up to 3 drinks per day does not seem to have an adverse effect on nerve or muscle, even in elderly people. Chronic alcoholics are definitely prone to neuropathy and myopathy, however.

Cognitive impairment is one of the most devastating complications of heavy drinking. The risk of developing dementia is increased in long-term alcoholics, and may be due to direct toxic effects of alcohol, thiamine deficiency, or a combination of these. Alcohol-related dementia appears to account for approximately 5% of dementias (Clarfield, 1988; Weytingh, 1995). Since it probably goes unrecognized quite often, the prevalence may actually be higher (Oslin, 2000). Several studies show an unusually high prevalence of alcoholism histories among people who carry a diagnosis of Alzheimer's Disease or nonspecified dementia. Men are somewhat more likely than women to have alcohol-related dementia, but as Mrs. M.'s case demonstrates, it is important to have a high index of suspicion for alcohol use disorders in all elderly people with cognitive impairment. (See chapter 3 by Atkinson and Misra on comorbidities for further information on this subject.)

Detecting alcohol problems in people with cognitive impairment is particularly important because alcoholism is probably one of the few truly reversible causes of dementia. In one study of 200 patients with dementia, only 2 patients had complete reversal of their cognitive impairment; one had dementia due to cimetidine and one to alcoholism (Larson, Barton, & Reifler, 1985). A meta-analysis of causes of dementia confirmed that alcoholism is one of the most common causes of potentially reversible dementia, accounting for around 4% of all dementia cases (Clarfield, 1988). The same report found that drugs and alcohol together, which they did not examine separately, were the causes of dementia most likely to reverse, either partly or completely. A more recent review of published studies found that 4.8% of partially or fully reversed dementias were due to alcohol (Weytingh, Bossuyt, & van Crevel,1995). An aggressive approach to alcoholism treatment is clearly worthwhile in people with alcohol-related dementia.

Heavy alcohol use affects other areas of neurologic functioning as well. Peripheral neuropathy, with paresthesias, pain, and weakness in the lower extremities is quite common and may interfere with mobility. Sometimes the upper extremities are also affected. Vitamin deficiencies probably play a role in the development of alcoholic neuropathy. This condition tends to be slowly progressive but may improve or resolve with alcohol cessation and a nutritious diet. Alcoholics may also develop autonomic neuropathy, with orthostatic hypotension and bladder or bowel dysfunction. People who consume very large amounts of alcohol are also prone to develop cerebellar degeneration, which causes truncal ataxia and often is accompanied by a wide-based gait. It is uncertain whether this condition develops in the absence of a thiamine deficiency. Around half of patients will improve when they stop drinking.

At high doses, alcohol is also toxic to muscle and chronic progressive muscle weakness is common in alcoholics. This tends to improve with abstinence from alcohol or even restricted alcohol use, but it appears that it does not often resolve completely.

The Gastrointestinal System

Mr. G. was a 72-year-old man who came to the emergency room at the Veterans Affairs Medical Center because of persistent vomiting for 2 days. Before that he had been in his usual state of health, which included fluctuating hypertension, intermittent paranoid delusions, and previous treatment for alcoholism. He was homeless and lived in shelters when the weather was bad. On exam, he was moderately unkempt and somnolent. Blood pressure was 120/60 lying down and dropped to 98/50 on standing, which caused him to become quite lightheaded. Abdominal exam was benign, but stool testing indicated occult bleeding from the gastrointestinal tract. He had a severe anemia with a hemoglobin of 7.6. Upper endoscopy showed erosive gastritis. He was treated with intravenous fluids, a blood transfusion, and omeprazole. He refused alcohol treatment and insisted on returning to his previous living situation when his medical condition stabilized.

Erosive gastritis is a common consequence of heavy drinking and is a common cause of upper gastrointestinal bleeding in alcoholics. Contrary to common belief, heavy alcohol use does not seem to increase the risk of peptic ulcer disease, though it may increase the risk of bleeding from ulcers (Aldoori et al., 1997). The patient described above also illustrates the phenomenon of coexisting chronic mental illness and alcoholism. Often in old age patients with this combination develop serious medical complications of their alcoholism and ultimately require nursing home care.

Alcohol also affects gastric and intestinal motility and causes histologic changes in intestinal mucosa. Gastric emptying is often delayed in alcoholics. Diarrhea and malabsorption are common consequences of heavy drinking in both chronic and binge drinkers. Malabsorption often contributes to the many nutritional deficiencies alcoholics are prone to, though poor diet is also often a factor.

Alcohol is directly toxic to the liver. The spectrum of liver disease caused by alcohol ranges from mild fatty infiltration to severe cirrhosis that can be fatal. The risk increases with both the amount consumed and the duration of use. However, there is a great deal of individual variation in susceptibility to alcoholic liver disease. Less than 30% of alcoholics develop cirrhosis, but some people develop it with as little as 2 drinks per day. Women are at risk of cirrhosis at about half the alcohol intake required to increase the risk for men (Becker, Deis, & Sorenson, 1996). Other factors, such as genetic susceptibility, exposure to hepatitis viruses, and exposure to hepatotoxic drugs also affect the risk of cirrhosis. Abstinence from alcohol improves survival in people with cirrhosis by about 20% in a five-year period. People with alcoholic cirrhosis who are over 60 years old have a higher one-year mortality rate than younger people with this condition.

The Cardiovascular System

Mr. M. was a loving and exemplary caregiver for his wife throughout her long course of Alzheimer's Disease. For the two years before her death, he was unable to care for her at home, but was an active volunteer at her nursing home and spent most of his days there caring for her and other residents. A few months after her death, Mr. M.'s hypertension, which had been quite mild and easily controlled, was no longer responsive to his medication. Increasing the dose and adding another medicine did not bring it under control. One day I thought to ask about his alcohol intake, which had always been moderate. It turned out that after his wife's death, Mr. M. had begun to visit a local bar almost daily for social contact. He had been consuming around 3 beers a day. I told him that this might be the reason his blood pressure was elevated and we discussed alternative strategies. He continued to go to the bar, but began to make every alternate drink nonalcoholic beer. The blood pressure returned to normal within a few weeks.

Hypertension is extremely prevalent among elderly people, affecting close to half of people 65 years and older. Since it is a major risk factor for stroke, myocardial infarction, and other adverse vascular events, it is extremely important that we control this condition. Several large epidemiologic studies have found a positive relationship between alcohol consumption and hypertension. The risk of high blood pressure is increased among people who consume 2 or more drinks per day and continues to increase with increasing levels of alcohol consumption (MacMahon, 1987). This is true for both men and women. Alcohol-related hypertension readily improves when alcohol consumption is decreased. Another important effect of alcohol for people with hypertension is its potential interaction with antihypertensive medications. A severe drop in blood pressure may occur acutely when alcohol is used concurrently with reserpine, methyldopa, hydralazine, nitroglycerine, and other antihypertensive or vasodilating drugs.

Many studies show that heavy drinking increases the risk of both ischemic and hemorrhagic stroke. A recent meta-analysis confirms this effect (Holman, English, Milne, & Winter, 1996) though some large well-done studies have not seen an increased risk (Thun et al., 1997). Moderate alcohol drinking, on the other hand, which many studies have found to protect against coronary disease (Gaziano et al., 1993; Rimm et al., 1991), may also have a protective effect for ischemic stroke (Sacco et al., 1999). Moderate drinking is thought to have much of its cardioprotective effect by favorably affecting lipids and preventing platelet aggregation. It may be that alcohol's beneficial effect on lipids and platelets competes with its adverse effect on blood pressure in the risk for stroke; it appears that heavy drinkers who also have hypertension are at the highest risk of stroke.

Long-term heavy drinkers are at risk of cardiomyopathy, which seems to be strongly related to lifetime alcohol intake. In women, cardiomyopathy occurs at lower levels of reported consumption (Fernandez-Sola et al., 1997). If this condition is recognized early, it can reverse with abstinence from alcohol, but more severe cardiomyopathy is less likely to improve. Cardiac arrhythmias are another complication of heavy drinking and seem to be most common among binge drinkers. Atrial fibrillation is the rhythm disturbance most commonly recognized, though ventricular arrhythmias have also been reported.

Cancer

Mr. A. was a 68-year-old insurance executive who had an increasingly hoarse voice over several months. He had discussed this with his physician, who advised him that it was not likely to be serious. Mr. A. had smoked briefly in young adulthood, but stopped when the health risks of smoking had been publicized in the 1960s. He had been a heavy social drinker for many years, with an average consumption of 3–5 drinks a day. Around a year after his initial visit to the doctor, Mr. A. noticed a lump on the side of his neck. When he went back to the doctor, it became evident that he had lost 15 pounds over that year as well. A biopsy of the lump showed cancer, which was coming from the larynx. Surgery was done, but the cancer recurred several months later and Mr. A. died from this disease a year after the diagnosis.

The risk of some cancers is increased among heavy drinkers. The evidence for this is clearest in the case of cancers of the head and neck. People who consume more than 2 alcoholic drinks per day have an increased risk of cancer of the mouth, pharynx, and larynx. The case of Mr. A. illustrates that symptoms such as hoarseness, that might indicate a cancer, should be pursued aggressively in heavy drinkers. The risk of head and neck cancers continues to rise with increasing levels of alcohol intake (Longnecker, 1995; Thun et al., 1997). Concurrent smoking further increases this risk; it is estimated that 75% of head and neck cancers are caused by alcohol, tobacco, or both. The risk of alcohol-related head and neck cancers is decreased somewhat, however, by a high intake of fruits and vegetables (Longnecker, 1995). The clinical course of cancers can also be affected by alcohol consumption. Among patients with head and neck cancers, mortality is higher among those who continue to drink heavily (Deleyiannis, Thomas, Vaughan, & Davis, 1996).

Many, but not all, studies show a relatively small increase in the risk of breast cancer in women who consume more than one drink per day and an increasing risk with larger amounts of alcohol consumption. In most studies, the risk is increased less than twofold among heavy drinkers (Longnecker, 1995). Some studies suggest that alcohol has less effect on the risk of breast cancer in postmenopausal women, but others show no decrease after menopause. Some have suggested that cumulative lifetime alcohol use is the most important factor. In others, current drinking seems to play a greater role. The questions of whether and how alcohol plays a causal or contributory role in the development of breast cancer remain a subject of intense investigation.

Heavy drinking increases the risk of esophageal cancer fivefold or more, a risk further increased by smoking. Alcohol also increases the risk of cancer of the liver, which is usually, but not always, preceded by cirrhosis in alcoholics. Concurrent viral hepatitis greatly increases the risk of liver cancer in alcoholics (Longnecker, 1995). For cancers of the colon, stomach, lung, and pancreas, data are conflicting. Heavy drinking does not appear to increase the risk of prostate cancer, the most common cancer among American men (Breslow & Weed, 1998).

Osteoporosis

Many elderly people suffer from consequences of osteoporosis. While this condition is more common in older women, men who live into their 80s and 90s are also at high risk for fractures due to osteoporosis. The role of alcohol in the development of osteoporosis is not clear. Alcohol does have direct suppressive effects on osteoblasts, and alcoholism clearly increases the risk of osteopenia in men (Rico, 1990). Since alcoholics are also prone to cigarette smoking, nutritional deficiencies, liver disease, and hypogonadism, however, the relative importance of each of these multiple risk factors is difficult to discern.

The relationship between moderate drinking and bone density seems to be complex. Slemenda studied male twins over a 16-year period and found that alcohol use was a strong predictor of decreased bone density over time, as was cigarette smoking. (Slemenda et al., 1992). Those who drank more than 1.5 drinks per day had nearly twice the rate of loss of abstainers. On the other hand, the Rancho Bernardo Study (Holbrook & Barrett-Conner, 1993) found that social drinking, even at 3 drinks a day, was associated with a small but statistically significant *increase* in bone mineral density 12 years later in both men and women. In the Framingham study also, elderly men and women who were heavy drinkers had higher bone density than light drinkers, though the effect was greater for women than men (Felson et al., 1995). Both of the latter studies were done in populations with relatively high socioeconomic status and good nutrition. A recent British study confirms a positive association between alcohol use and bone density (Dennison et al., 1999). One possible proposed mechanism for this effect is an alcohol-related increase in estrogen level. Though the effect of endogenous estrogen on bone density in men has not been extensively explored, there is some evidence that it plays a role in age-related bone loss in men. The current state of knowledge suggests that alcohol use is a risk factor for significant osteopenia only with very high levels of consumption and perhaps only when associated with nutritional deficiencies.

Falls

Several studies have examined risk factors for falls and found alcohol either not to be associated with or to be protective against falls (Tinetti,

Speechley, & Ginter, 1988; Nevitt, Cummings, Kidd, & Black, 1989; O'Loughlin, Robitaille, Boivin, & Suissa, 1993). However, a large prospective study from Finland examined risk factors for fall-related injuries that caused hospitalization or death (Malmivaara et al., 1993). Among 19,518 persons followed for 8–11 years, 628 such injuries occurred. The risk of injurious falls increased with increasing level of alcohol intake in all age groups. Those 65 and older who consumed 1,000 g per month (about 23 drinks per week) or more had a statistically significant risk that was 8 times that of abstainers. The difference between these studies may be due largely to the sample size and the selection of subjects. Moderately heavy drinkers with good nutrition probably do not suffer adverse effects on nerve, bone, or muscle. Indeed, some studies suggest better strength and mobility among moderate drinkers (Lacroix et al., 1993; Nelson et al., 1994). Population-based studies, such as the one from Finland, have a sufficient number of *very* heavy drinkers to show adverse effects. Most other studies have recruited volunteers, who are more likely to be moderate drinkers with good nutrition and health status.

Hip fracture is of particular concern, since it is such a devastating consequence of falls for older people. Though some studies have shown a positive association between alcohol use and hip fracture, especially in middle-aged people, the majority of well done prospective studies of elderly people do not (Hemenway, Azrael, Rimm, Feskanich, & Willet, 1994; Mussolino, Looker, Madans, Langlois, & Orwoll, 1998; Cummings et al., 1995; Grisso et al., 1991) It appears that, as in the case of cardiovascular disease, alcohol may have both beneficial and adverse effects. Whether alcohol use contributes to hip fractures in a given group or individual probably depends on the amount consumed, the pattern of drinking (steady vs. binge drinking), the nutritional state, health status, age, and other factors.

Medication Interactions

Mr. Y. was a 76-year-old man who had had an aortic valve replacement. He had an excellent result from the surgery, but required lifelong anticoagulation therapy to prevent embolic events. Mr. Y. had been a lifelong "heavy social drinker." His warfarin requirements varied widely from time to time and it became evident that he was consuming large amounts of alcohol at somewhat irregular intervals. After we discussed the interaction between alcohol and warfarin, Mr. Y. attempted to decrease his alcohol intake and avoid binges. He was not able to maintain this for long periods of time, so we discussed possible alcohol treatment programs to help him abstain from alcohol use altogether. He was unwilling to do this and several months later, despite intensive monitoring of his anticoagulation, he was hospitalized with severe gastrointestinal bleeding.

Alcohol is used concurrently with medications by a large number of elderly people. Many of these medications have potential to interact adversely with alcohol, though studies that investigate actual clinical outcomes are sparse. Heavy alcohol consumption probably increases the risk most substantially, but even light or moderate drinking can be problematic when alcohol is consumed concurrently with certain medications.

One reason potential drug-alcohol interactions are important for elderly people is simply the high frequency of medication use in this population. At least 75% of people 65 and older use some medication and around half use 3 or more medications. The number of medications taken is itself an important risk factor for adverse drug reactions. Since alcohol has many effects on various organ systems, we must consider it a "drug." Simply consuming alcohol in effect adds another drug to one's medication profile. Many people do add this particular drug: at least 50% of older people consume some alcohol. One cannot assume that older people abstain from alcohol when they are taking medications. In one study of elderly (mean age 83) retirement community residents in Wisconsin, 77% used medications, 47% used alcohol, and 38% concurrently used alcohol and medications with a strong potential for adverse interactions (Adams, 1995a). There are many ways alcohol may interact with medications (Adams, 1995b). Here we will discuss altered drug levels, central nervous system depression, and bleeding.

Altered Drug Levels

Most alcohol is metabolized in the liver by an enzyme called alcohol dehydrogenase (ADH). Regular heavy alcohol use increases the activity of this enzyme, which increases the rate at which alcohol is metabolized. Alcohol can also increase, or "induce," other drug metabolizing enzymes in the liver. The increased enzyme activity then causes more rapid breakdown of drugs. Because the drugs are being rapidly broken down, the patient develops lower blood levels. Some of the important medications affected by enzyme induction are the anticoagulant warfarin, the antiseizure drug phenytoin, the sedative diazepam and other benzodiazepines, the antihypertensive propranolol, and the antimicrobial isoniazid.

In contrast to the enzyme induction cause by chronic heavy drinking, *short term* heavy alcohol use has an essentially opposite effect on drug metabolism. When a large amount of alcohol is ingested acutely, the enzyme system is occupied by the alcohol and is not as available for drug metabolism. Less of the drug is broken down, and higher blood levels result. Warfarin, diazepam, and isoniazid, as well as many other drugs, are affected by this phenomenon. Since long-term heavy alcohol use causes increased metabolism and short-term alcohol use causes decreased metabolism of some of the same drugs, prescribing for heavy drinkers can be a nightmare for clinicians. Safe use of anticoagulants and antiseizure medications can be close to impossible for patients who abuse alcohol.

ADH also occurs in the stomach. Several studies have shown inhibition of gastric alcohol dehydrogenase by cimetidine, ranitidine, and nizatidine, causing blood alcohol levels 30%–40% higher than would be seen after an equal amount of alcohol alone. Even in the absence of these drugs, elderly people develop higher blood alcohol levels than younger people by mechanisms discussed above. A further increase due to an interaction with one of these drugs may cause an unwitting elderly person to experience unexpectedly severe effects from a moderate amount of alcohol intake. While there is clearly potential for this interaction to lead to such adverse outcomes as falls or automobile accidents, the clinical importance of this effect has not been studied.

Central Nervous System Depression

Susceptibility to the effects of drugs that suppress central nervous system activity, such as benzodiazepines, narcotics and antihistamines, increases with age. These drugs often cause increased sedation in elderly people. There is also an increased risk of falls among elderly people using long-acting benzodiazepines, which implies an increased sensitivity to the CNS effects of these drugs. Concurrent use of benzodiazepines and other agents that suppress central nervous system functions may impair balance and predispose to falls, cause slower reaction times and lead to an automobile accident, or cause excessive sleepiness. Alcohol, which has CNS depressant effects, has an added sedative effect when combined with these drugs. The combination is well known to cause serious impairment of the motor skills and judgment needed for driving, operating machinery, and many other activities.

Psychotropic drugs are most likely to produce this effect. Benzodiazepines in particular are used very commonly by elderly people and have strong potential for this type of interaction. Both sedation and impairment of the skills needed for driving have been documented and have potential to cause serious adverse outcomes for elderly people. Some tricyclic antidepressants also interact with alcohol to impair alertness and motor functioning; amitriptyline and nortriptyline are the best studied. Most studies of the CNS effects of drug-alcohol combinations have been done on healthy young subjects. Since elderly people are more susceptible to the effects of some benzodiazepines and are more likely to have illnesses that predispose them to adverse effects of drugs, it is probable that older people are even more likely than the subjects of most studies to experience adverse drug-alcohol interactions of this sort. Further research is needed to define the specifics of these effects. However, enough is known that physicians should advise their patients taking CNS depressant drugs to abstain from alcohol. Patients using CNS depressant drugs should particularly be told not to drive a motor vehicle if concurrent use should occur.

Bleeding

Arthritis and other musculoskeletal problems are among the most common problems for which older people consult physicians. Nonsteroidal anti-inflammatory drugs (NSAIDs) and aspirin are very commonly prescribed or recommended for the treatment of these disorders. The effects of NSAIDs alone on the GI tract appear to be more severe in older people. When older people do have gastrointestinal bleeding, they are more likely to die from it than younger people. When NSAIDs and aspirin are used concurrently with alcohol, they cause longer bleeding times, increased gastric inflammation, and an increased risk of gastrointestinal bleeding (Kaufman, 1999). Since gastritis and gastrointestinal bleeding are common complications of alcoholism as well as of NSAID use, the risk is particularly high in alcoholics. This interaction may, however, occur with moderate drinking as well.

Bleeding can also occur as a result of interaction between alcohol and warfarin. Warfarin dosing, as illustrated in the case of Mr. Y., can be extremely difficult when a patient is drinking alcohol. The risk of serious bleeding is particularly high in alcoholics (McMahan, Smith, Carey, & Zhou, 1998). This interaction occurs because of the effects of alcohol and the medication on liver enzymes. In the case of chronic heavy drinking, metabolism of the drug in the liver is increased and lower blood levels of the drug are acquired. Higher doses are required to achieve the desired effect. The effect may persist up to weeks after cessation of alcohol use, so careful attention to changes in dose requirements is needed for a long period of time. Since many people move in and out of heavy drinking status over time, physicians must be constantly alert to the changing potential for drug-alcohol interactions in these patients. These problems and others related to fluctuating drug requirements by heavy drinkers can only be prevented by counseling patients about the potential interactions and by vigilance on the part of the prescribing physician.

Liver Toxicity

Another result of enzyme induction by long-term heavy alcohol use is the increased production of metabolites toxic to the liver during the breakdown of certain drugs (Lieber, 1991). Some of the most notable examples of this effect are the hepatotoxicity of isoniazid, phenylbutazone, and acetaminophen. An alcoholic who sprains an ankle, unaware of the potential liver toxicity from the combination of alcohol and acetaminophen, may take relatively large doses of this drug for pain. Severe liver necrosis can result. Since acetaminophen is easily available over the counter, appropriate labeling and public education are needed to warn people about this potentially life-threatening combination. Alcoholics have an increased susceptibility to tuberculosis and isoniazid is commonly used to treat it. This combination may also be highly toxic to the liver. Patients who may be heavy drinkers must be monitored especially carefully for elevations of liver enzymes while using these drugs.

Because of these and other potential drug-alcohol interactions, discussing possible interactions with alcohol should be a regular part of educating patients about their medicines.

Summary

Heavy alcohol use is clearly detrimental to health. Older people are somewhat less likely than younger people to drink heavily, but those who do are at least as susceptible to adverse consequences. Indeed, Medicare is billed for alcohol-related hospitalizations among elderly people as commonly as for acute myocardial infarction (Adams, Yuan, Barboriak, & Rimm, 1993). It is incumbent on health care professionals to ask patients about their alcohol use and to intervene when it puts them at risk for health problems. Many of the health problems discussed in this chapter are caused by moderately heavy drinking, in the range of 3–4 drinks per day. Brief cognitive behavioral interventions in the primary care setting are very successful with these moderately heavy drinkers (Fleming et al., 1999). People who are dependent on alcohol are often helped by more intensive treatment programs and 12-step groups. Older people successfully complete treatment at least as often as younger people and should always be referred when appropriate.

References

Adams, W. L. (1995a). Potential for adverse drug-alcohol interactions in elderly retirement community residents. *Journal of the American Geriatric Society, 43,* 1021–1025.

Adams, W. L. (1995b). Interactions between alcohol and medications. *International Journal of Addictions, 30,* 1679–1699.

Adams, W. L., Yuan, Z., Barboriak, J. J., & Rimm, A. A. (1993). Alcohol-related hospitalizations in elderly people: Prevalence and geographic variation in the United States. *Journal of the American Medical Association, 270,* 1222–1225.

Aldoori, W. H., Giovannucci, E. L., Stampfer, M. J., Rimm, E. B., Wing, A. L., & Willett, W. C. (1997). A prospective study of alcohol, smoking, caffeine, and the risk of duodenal ulcer in men. *Epidemiology, 8,* 420–424.

Becker, U., Deis, A., Sorenson, T. I. A., Gronbaek, M., Borch-Johnson, K., Muller, C. F., Schnohr, P., & Jensen, G. (1996). Prediction of the risk of liver disease by alcohol intake, sex and age: A prospective population study. *Hepatology, 23,* 1025–1029.

Breslow, R. A., & Weed, D. L. (1998). Review of epidemiologic studies of alcohol and prostate cancer. *Nutritional Cancer, 30,* 1–13.

Clarfield, A. M. (1988). The reversible dementias: Do they reverse? *Annals of Internal Medicine, 109,* 476–486.

Cummings, S. R., Nevitt, M. C., Browner, W. S., Stone, K., Fox, K. M., Ensrud, K. E., Cauley, J. C., Black, D., & Vogt, T. M. (1995). Risk factors for hip fracture in white women. *New England Journal of Medicine, 332,* 767–773.

Deleyiannis, F. W., Thomas, D. B., Vaughan, T. L., & Davis, S. (1996). Alcoholism: Independent predictor of survival in patients with head and neck cancer. *Journal of National Cancer Institute, 88,* 542–549.

Dennison, E., Eastell, R., Fall, C. H., Kellingray, S., Wood, P. H., & Cooper, C. (1999). Determinants of bone loss in elderly men and women: A prospective population-based study. *Osteoporosis International, 10*(5), 384–391.

Felson, D. T., Kiel, D. P., Anderson, J. J., & Kannel, W. B. (1988). Alcohol consumption and hip fractures: The Framingham study. *American Journal of Epidemiology, 128,* 1102–1110.

Felson, D. T., Zhang, Y. A., Hannan, M. T., Kannel, W. B., & Kiel, D. P. (1995). Alcohol intake and bone-mineral density in elderly men and women: The Framingham Study. *American Journal of Epidemiology, 142*(5), 485–492.

Fernandez-Sola, J., Estruch, R., Nicolas, J. M., Pare, J. C., Sacanella, E., Antunez, E., & Urbano-Marquez, A. (1997). Comparison of alcoholic cardiomyopathy in women versus men. *American Journal of Cardiology, 80,* 481–485.

Fernandez-Sola, J., Nicolas, J. M., Sacanella, E., Robert, J., Cofan, R. J., Estruch, R., & Urbano-Marquez, A. (2000). Low-dose ethanol consumption allows strength recovery in chronic alcoholic myopathy. *Quarterly Journal of Medicine, 93*(1), 35–40.

Fleming, M. F., Barry, K. L., Manwell, L., Adams, W. L., Stauffacher, E. A. (1999). Brief physician advice for alcohol problems in older adults: A randomized community-based trial. *American Journal of Family Practice, 48,* 378–384.

Gaziano, J. M., Buring, J. E., Breslow, J. L., Goldhaber, S. Z., Rosner, B., Vandenburgh, M., Willett, W., & Hennekens, C. H. (1993). Moderate alcohol intake, increased levels of high-density lipoprotein and its subfractions, and decreased risk of myocardial infarction. *New England Journal of Medicine, 329,* 1829–1834.

Grisso, J. A., Kelsey, J. L., Strom, B., Chiu, G. Y., Maislin, G., O'Brien, L. A., Hoffman, S., & Kaplan, F. (1991). Risk factors for falls as a cause of hip fracture in women. *New England Journal of Medicine, 324,* 1326–1331.

Hemenway, D., Azrael, D. R., Rimm, E. B., Feskanich, D., & Willet, W. C. (1994). Risk factors for hip fracture in U.S. men aged 40 through 75 years. *American Journal of Public Health, 84,* 1843–1845.

Hernandez-Munoz, R., Caballeria, J., Baraona, E., Uppal, R., Greenstein, R., & Lieber, C. S. (1990). Human gastric alcohol dehydrogenase: Its inhibition by H2–receptor antagonists and its effect on the bioavailability of ethanol. *Alcoholism, Clinical and Experimental Research, 14,* 946–950.

Holbrook, T. L., & Barrett-Conner, E. (1993). A prospective study of alcohol consumption and bone mineral density. *British Medical Journal, 306,* 1506–1509.

Holman, C. D. J., English, D. R., Milne, E., & Winter, M. G. (1996). Meta-analysis of alcohol and all-cause mortality: A validation of NHMRC recommendations. *Medical Journal of Australia, 164,* 141–145.

Kaufman, D. W., Kelly, J. P., Wiholm, B. E., Laszlo, A., Sheehan, J. E., Koff, R. S., & Shapiro, S. (1999). The risk of acute major upper gastrointestinal bleeding among users of aspirin and ibuprofen at various levels of alcohol consumption. *American Journal of Gastroenterology, 94,* 3189–3196.

LaCroix, A. Z., Guralnik, J. M., Berkman, L. F., Wallace, R. B., & Satterfield, S. (1993). Maintaining mobility in late life II: Smoking, alcohol consumption, physical activity, and body mass index. *American Journal of Epidemiology, 137,* 858–869.

Larson, E. B., Burton, V., & Reifler B. (1985). Diagnostic evaluation of 200 elderly outpatients with suspected dementia. *Journal of Gerontology, 40,* 536–543.

Lieber, C. S. (1991). Hepatic, metabolic and toxic effects of ethanol: 1991 update. *Alcoholism: Clinical and Experimental Research, 15,* 573–592.

Longnecker, M. P. (1995). Alcohol consumption and risk of cancer in humans: An overview. *Alcohol, 12,* 87–96.

MacMahon, S. (1987). Alcohol consumption and hypertension. *Hypertension, 9,* 111–112.

Malmivaara, A., Heliovaara, M., Knekt, P., Reunanen, A., & Aromaa, A. (1993). Risk factors for injurious falls leading to hospitalization or death in a cohort of 19,500 adults. *American Journal of Epidemiology, 138,* 384–394.

McMahan, D. A., Smith, D. M., Carey, M. A., & Zhou, X. H. (1998). Risk of major hemorrhage for outpatients treated with warfarin. *Journal of General Internal Medicine, 13*(5), 311–316.

Mussolino, M. E., Looker, A. C., Madans, J. H., Langlois, J. A., & Orwoll, E. S. (1998). Risk factors for hip fracture in white men: The NHANES I epidemiologic follow-up study. *Journal of Bone and Mineral Research, 13,* 918–924.

Nelson, H. D., Nevitt, M. C., Scott, J. C., Stone, K. L., & Cummings, S. R. (1994). Smoking, alcohol, and neuromuscular and physical function of older women. *Journal of the American Medical Association, 272,* 1825–1831.

Nevitt, M. C., Cummings, S. R., Kidd, S., & Black, D. (1989). Risk factors for recurrent nonsyncopal falls. *Journal of the American Medical Association, 261,* 2663–2668.

O'Loughlin, J. L., Robitaille, Y., Boivin, J. F., & Suissa, S. (1993). Incidence of and risk factors for falls and injurious falls among the community-dwelling elderly. *American Journal of Epidemiology, 137,* 342–354.

Oslin, D. (2000). Alcohol use in late life—disability and comorbidity. *Journal of Geriatric Psychiatry and Neurology, 13*(3), 134–140.

Oslin, D., Atkinson, R. M., Smith, D. M., & Hendrie, H. (1998). Alcohol related dementia: proposed clinical criteria. *International Journal of Geriatric Psychiatry, 13*(4), 203–212.

Rico, H. (1990). Alcohol and bone disease. *Alcohol and Alcoholism, 25,* 345–352.

Rimm, E. B., Giovannucci, E. L., Willett, W. C., Colditz, G. A., Ascherio, A., Rosner, B., & Stampfer, M. J. (1991). Prospective study of alcohol consumption and risk of coronary disease in men. *The Lancet, 338,* 464–468.

Sacco, R. L., Elkind, M., Boden-Albala, B., Lin, I. F., Kargman, D. E., Hauser, W. A., Shea, S., & Paik, M. C. (1999). The protective effects of moderate alcohol consumption on ischemic stroke. *Journal of the American Medical Association, 281,* 53–60.

Slemenda, C. W., Christian, J. C., Reed, T., Reister, T. K., Williams, C. J., & Jonston, C. C. (1992). Long-term bone loss in men: Effects of genetic and environmental factors. *Annals of Internal Medicine, 117,* 286–291.

Thun, M. J., Peto, R., Lopez, A. D., Monaco, J. H., Henley, S. J., Heath, C. W., & Doll, R. (1997). Alcohol consumption and mortality among middle-aged and elderly U.S. adults. *New England Journal of Medicine, 337,* 1705–1714.

Tinetti, M. E., Speechley, M., & Ginter, S. F. (1988). Risk factors for falls among elderly persons living in the community. *New England Journal of Medicine, 319,* 1701–1707.

Weytingh, M. D., Bossuyt, P. M., & van Crevel, H. (1995). Reversible dementia: More than 10% or less than 1%? A quantitative review. *Journal of Neurology, 242,* 466–471.

4

Mental Disorders and Symptoms in Older Alcoholics

Roland M. Atkinson and Sahana Misra

A Brief History of Psychiatric Comorbidity

Until just a few years ago, symptoms of depression and anxiety in alcoholics were usually considered to be part of the disorder of alcoholism. For narrative ease, we will use the terms "alcohol use disorders," "problem drinking," and "alcoholism" interchangeably. Each term has its own definition, of course, and we have offered definitions elsewhere (Atkinson, 2000). But in clinical practice—among the older adults referred for treatment—there is in fact a great deal of overlap, i.e., most problem drinkers also meet criteria for a DSM-IV alcohol use disorder (American Psychiatric Association, 1994) and would be called alcoholic according to the most recent definition of that term (Morse and Flavin, 1992). For other mental disorders we have followed the terminology of DSM-IV throughout. Clients in substance abuse treatment tended to receive the same care whether they complained of such symptoms or not. Staff were untrained in the diagnosis or treatment of mental disorders. Alcoholics with obvious major mental disorders were not accepted into alcoholism treatment and instead were trundled off to the psychiatric clinic. These were the "dark ages" with respect to our understanding of psychiatric comorbidity and its relevance to clients' treatment needs.

This began to change after 1980, when improved diagnostic guidelines were created for psychiatric and substance use disorders, and clinicians were encouraged for the first time to specify *all* disorders which a given patient might be suffering from, rather than attempt to explain all the findings on the basis of a single diagnosis. Door-to-door community surveys followed, based on the use of these new guidelines, and these surveys demonstrated that large numbers of people suffered from both substance-related and other psychiatric disorders. For example, someone with an alcohol use disorder who also met the new criteria for a diagnosis of a major depressive disorder could be said to suffer from a coexisting or *comorbid* depressive disorder. Patients with substance use disorders who also suffer from comorbid psychiatric disorders are often referred to as having *"dual diagnoses."*

At about this time other studies began to show that when clients in substance treatment programs who had persistent mental symptoms were treated by counselors trained in mental health practices, they responded more favorably than clients with high levels of emotional distress who received traditional counseling from staff who only had knowledge of substance abuse. The importance of psychiatric comorbidity and its revelance to adequate, properly individualized treatment gradually became recognized.

Some Concepts and Definitions

The earlier approach—trying to fit all the mental symptoms into the sole diagnosis of alcoholism—wasn't entirely wrong. Newly admitted alcoholics who have been drinking heavily for weeks or months tend to be depressed. If treated conservatively (with adequate medications for detoxification; attention to hydration, diet, vitamin and mineral replacement; treatment of medical problems as needed; and consistent interactions with a calm and reassuring staff), depressive symptoms—even when they meet criteria for major depression—resolve *spontaneously* in the majority of cases within about 3 to 4 weeks, without any need for specific antidepressant treatment (Brown & Schuckit, 1988; Brown et al., 1995). Depression of this type is termed an *alcohol-induced* mood disorder, and, because it is an ephemeral—a transient—complication of alcoholic levels of drinking, it is not considered a true, comorbid depressive disorder. The same can be said for many anxiety symptoms that distress alcohol-dependent patients during withdrawal.

But when depression, anxiety, or other symptoms persist more or less unchanged for weeks or longer after drinking has ceased, or occur during prolonged abstinent intervals, and these symptoms meet criteria for diagnosis of a mental disorder, then one can be sure that a comorbid disorder actually exists. This distinction is clinically important, because it is well known that whatever diagnoses patients are labeled with often influence how they are treated for years to come. Comorbid disorders can be either independent (the cause has nothing to do with alcoholism—for example, schizophrenia) or alcohol induced (for example, alcohol-induced persisting amnesic disorder or alcohol-induced persisting dementia).

Two other terms tend to add confusion in discussions of comorbidity: "primary" and "secondary." These terms are used by epidemiologists, in cases where two disorders coexist in a patient's life history, to specify which disorder occurred first. The earlier disorder is termed *primary,* the later one *secondary.* For example, if the earliest symptoms of alcohol dependence occurred when a patient was 42, and the first symptoms of major depression occurred at age 50, then the alcohol dependence is considered primary and depression, secondary. Unfortunately these terms imply causal relationships when there may be no evidence whatsoever to substantiate this. The primary disorder is not necessarily the cause of the secondary disorder in this context, although it might be.

Another term that has become fashionable lately is "subsyndromal." When, for example, depressive symptoms are present and cause dysfunction, but they fail to meet the criteria required for a diagnosis of one of the depressive disorders, the illness may be labeled *subsyndromal* depression. There is increasing evidence that symptoms in such cases may respond to the same treatments that benefit full-blown disorders. This is true, for example, in subsyndromal depression in the elderly. Finally, it is entirely possible in clinical practice—in fact it is quite common—to encounter alcoholic patients who have true comorbid depression or anxiety aggravated further by alcohol-induced symptoms. So the clinical picture at initial assessment may represent a composite in which the symptoms have more than a single cause.

Psychiatric Comorbidity in Older Adults

In a VA study that used national data, Blow and his coworkers showed that among military veterans seeking treatment for alcohol use disorders, the proportion who have comorbid psychiatric disorders remains quite high across the adult life span: about 50% of alcoholics in every age group had comorbid mental disorders (Blow, Cook, Booth, Falcon & Friedman 1992). Beginning in 1988, a number of published reports from various single-site programs have also documented the prevalence and types of comorbid psychiatric disorders seen in older adult problem drinkers (these are summarized in Atkinson, 1998). These studies show that about 30% to 60% of older alcoholics suffer from at least one comorbid psychiatric disorder. So the problem of comorbidity is as substantial in the older population as it is in younger groups.

Depressive mood disorders, dementias and subsyndromal cognitive deficits, and anxiety disorders are the most commonly documented mental disorders, accounting for perhaps 75% to 80% of all psychiatric comorbidity found in older alcoholics.* Because of their prominence, we will focus on these three groups of comorbid conditions in the remainder of this chapter.

Depression

Depression and alcohol use disorders are strongly linked across the life span, and this comorbid association persists into later life (see Atkinson, 1999, for a more extensive discussion of the relationship among depression, alcoholism, and aging). Depressive disorders include major depression, dysthymic disorder, adjustment disorder with depressed mood, alcohol-induced depression, and a few other conditions. The symptoms in all of these disorders are similar, varying only in number, severity and context for different diagnoses.

There is no convincing evidence that depression causes alcoholism. But in persons with well established alcoholic drinking patterns, the presence of depression often influences drinking behavior: self-medication for negative emotions is undoubtedly common in older alcoholics. For example, Dupree asked 214 older alcoholics how they felt *before* taking their first drink on a typical drinking day (Dupree & Schonfeld, 1998). A great majority reported feeling depressed, lonely, sad, bored, withdrawn, or other negative affects, but when asked how they felt *after*

*Schizophrenic, bipolar, and personality disorders account for most of the other cases. Alcohol, or alcohol withdrawal, can induce a number of acute psychiatric conditions apart from depression, anxiety, or cognitive impairment, including psychotic and sleep disorders, but these are seen primarily during and briefly following detoxification (American Psychiatric Association, 1994).

their first drink, 70% reported positive feelings. There is also evidence that among older nonproblem drinkers, those with an established pattern of increasing their drinking in response to negative affects or stress ("reactive" drinking pattern) are at greater risk for subsequently developing subsyndromal alcohol-related problems (Schutte, Brennan & Moos, 1998).

Although a few drinks can act temporarily as self-medication to assuage depressed feelings, this is a transient effect, lasting only for a few hours. The cumulative effects of a pattern of regular excessive alcohol consumption will typically lead to a worsening of an active bout of depression (Atkinson, 1999). Heavy drinking by alcoholics can also induce depression in persons who have no underlying comorbid depressive disorder. Alcohol-induced depression is detectible in perhaps half of all newly hospitalized alcoholics who have been drinking heavily up to the time of admission, and tends to run its course in about 1 to 3 weeks, remitting without the need for antidepressant medication (Brown et al., 1995). Many cases are subsyndromal, but others can become severe enough to meet criteria for major depression. Here is an illustrative case:

Case 1: Alcohol Dependence With Alcohol-Induced Depression. BD, a 65-year-old former stockbroker, was admitted to the general psychiatry unit for depression, suicidal thinking and "forgetfulness." He had been a heavy drinker since his teens, resulting in "blackouts" as early as age 13, military court martial for drunken disorderly conduct at 18, and, in later adulthood, falls resulting in injury, business failures, and a divorce. He had never been treated for alcoholism. He had a self-limited, untreated depressive episode at age 39 following an alcohol-related business failure.

At age 63 he had been forced to retire and began drinking more because of "boredom." His second spouse then left him for another man. Despondent over these developments, he drank even more and became progressively depressed over a 3-month period, with sleep decreased to 3–4 hours/night, loss of appetite, a 5-pound weight loss, and emerging plans to kill himself by drowning. Several paternal uncles, all four siblings, and an adult son are all alcoholic, but there is no family history of depression.

On admission he rated his mood as 9, with 10 being the worst depression he had ever felt. Although he received no specific antidepressant treatment, within 5 days he no longer thought of suicide, and his sleep and mood had improved substantially. Four weeks after admission, his score on the depression scale of the Minnesota Multiphasic Personality Inventory (MMPI) was normal (*T* score 56).

After engaging successfully in a supportive group therapy program for older alcoholics, he remained abstinent over the next year and stabilized his social circumstances. Depression did not reoccur, and his early subjective complaint of forgetfulness also waned. After a year of sobriety his score on the Mini-Mental State Examination (MMSE) was 26/30.

Case Discussion. This man with longstanding alcoholism was vulnerable to increased drinking problems when faced with life stressors in his 60s. Although depressive symptoms were probably induced by a combination of losses and alcohol effects, the sequence of events, especially the spontaneous relief of his depression within a few days of ceasing alcohol use, suggests alcohol-induced depression, and *not* a comorbid major depressive disorder. His transient forgetfulness was probably multifactorial, caused both by his alcohol use and depression. Abstinence from alcohol and peer social support, rather than antidepressant treatment, have determined his favorable course.

True comorbid depression, unlike alcohol-induced depression, lasts beyond a few weeks of sobriety or occurs during prolonged abstinent intervals. Comorbid depressive disorders are reported to be present in 9% to 28% of older alcoholics. Here is a case in point:

Case 2: Alcohol Dependence With Comorbid Major Depressive Disorder. IC, a 69-year-old recently divorced homemaker, was admitted to the medical service after being found unconscious at home. Her blood alcohol level was very high, 332 mg/100 ml. She gradually regained consciousness and had an uncomplicated recovery with supportive medical care. She had drunk table wine regularly throughout adulthood, up to a gallon per week, consuming more whenever confronted by stress, anxiety or depressive symptoms. Consumption had escalated even further in the past few months after she was divorced by her husband of 46 years. Always dependent upon others, she feared she could not look after herself and said she drank more to assuage her fear and despair, until she "lost control." She had, over the last 15 years, also solicited and overused prescribed benzodiazepines and codeine-containing analgesic medications for a variety of minor emotional and physical complaints. She had received various antidepressant medications over the past several years, but had never been hospitalized for psychiatric problems. Family history was negative for alcoholism and mood disorder.

On the ward her mental status was not remarkable after recovery from alcohol-induced coma, which was judged not to be a suicidal act, but rather the consequence of a drinking binge. She joined and sustained her involvement in Alcoholics Anonymous (AA), and has remained abstinent from alcohol for nearly 5 years. She also gradually was weaned from longstanding daily low doses of two benzodiazepine antianxiety medications, chlorazepate and triazolam.

However, 2 years after her hospitalization, she still had not adapted to living alone and developed symptoms of major depression. She was admitted to a general psychiatry inpatient unit where she responded well to an antidepressant medication, doxepin. Thereafter she continued to take antidepressants on a maintenance basis and, during regular supportive individual psychotherapy, was encouraged to live more independently. After three years she has not had a depressive relapse, was able to attend her granddaughter's wedding 1,000 miles away, and recently journeyed on a vacation trip to France.

Case discussion. It is not clear in this woman's history whether alcohol dependence or depressive episodes occurred first (i.e., which was primary and which secondary). But it is apparent that, unlike the situation in the first case, a major depressive episode arose after a lengthy period of abstinence. Alcohol excess could not be implicated in the etiology of this episode, and specific antidepressant treatment was necessary. The negative family history of depression is somewhat unusual, although many people lack information about mental illness in their relatives. She clearly had a comorbid depressive disorder. Her lifelong pattern of increasing her drinking in reaction to stress and emotional symptoms undoubtedly put her at risk for further alcohol-related problems. There is evidence that patients who regularly take benzodiazepines over long periods of time actually have increased levels of anxiety and depression as a result. Weaning off these medications may also have helped her achieve greater emotional stability. Her positive engagement in AA attests to the usefulness of this path to recovery for some elderly alcoholics.

As mentioned earlier, drinking may aggravate a preexisting comorbid depression, i.e., alcohol-induced symptoms may be superimposed during an episode of comorbid depression, so that the course of depressive symptoms is less clear-cut once drinking ceases. This complex situation is illustrated by the next case:

Case 3: Alcohol Dependence With Mixed Comorbid and Alcohol-Induced Depression. HG, a 65-year-old retired geologist, entered the general psychiatric unit because of gradually increasing depression and suicidal impulses after his spouse divorced him, persuading him in the process to consent to a settlement that also left him homeless and financially impoverished. He had begun heavy daily drinking in his 30s, but after two DUI convictions and threatened divorce, he entered alcoholism treatment at age 53 and remained abstinent for several years. Later, however, he resumed social drinking, then gradually escalated his daily consumption, and re-entered alcoholism treatment a few months ago. He was sober for "100 days" but then began to feel depressed, resuming heavy alcohol use to combat his low moods, and thus provoking his spouse's decision to divorce him.

Bouts of depression had begun at puberty, and through the years he had experienced frequent prolonged periods of depression in response to idleness, work pressures, marital conflict, and excessive drinking. There was no family history of alcoholism or mood disorder.

On the psychiatric unit he received no antidepressant medication, but over the first few days he nevertheless showed considerable improvement in mood and energy level, with disappearance of his suicidal preoccupation. He then was able to participate effectively in a 30-day residential alcoholism treatment program. When evaluated for possible acceptance into an outpatient group treatment program for older problem drinkers, 45 days after his last drink, and still not receiving antidepressant medication, he displayed appropriate, flexible affect and behavior, had no suicidal thoughts, but did have an underlying mood of sadness and expressed regrets about his losses. At that time his score on the Depression scale of the MMPI was highly elevated (*T* score 98), consistent with clinical depression. Effective management included enrollment in a homeless domiciliary program, age-specific alcoholism group treatment, and antidepressant medication.

Case Discussion. This man's longstanding vulnerability to depression predated the first manifestations of his alcohol dependence disorder and was consistent with a diagnosis of a (comorbid) dysthymic disorder. Depression is considered the primary disorder, with alcohol dependence secondary, since depressive problems began earlier in life. When he entered the psychiatric unit, his suicidal depressive state rapidly improved but without complete resolution. In fact, he was still clinically depressed after more than 6 weeks of sobriety and psychosocial assistance. The early partial improvement in his depression is attributable to alcohol-induced depressive effects, which abated, while the lingering symptoms represent his persisting symptomatic dysthymic disorder that required antidepressant treatment. Research shows that one predictor of persisting depression in recently detoxified alcoholics is major unresolved life problems, which this man obviously faced in abundance.

Table 4.1 Alcohol-Induced Depression Versus Comorbid Depression[a]

Feature	Alcohol-Induced Depression	Comorbid (Persistent) Depression
May meet criteria for major depression	+	+
Prior episodes occurred while drinking	+	+
Begins to improve after just a few days' sobriety	+	–
May take 2–3 weeks to resolve if untreated	+	–
Tends to persist more than 3 weeks if untreated	–	+
First episode may have predated alcohol problems	–	+
Prior episodes occurred during abstinent periods	–	+
Family history of depression/suicide more likely	–	+
Current major life problems/stressors more likely	–	+

Note. Based on Atkinson, 1999; Brown et al., 1995. Adapted with permission.
[a]The two conditions may co-occur (see text)

Differential Diagnosis and Treatment

In Table 4.1 we have attempted to list some guidelines that may help clinicians to distinguish between alcohol-induced and comorbid depression in recently drinking alcoholics. Experts do not agree on how soon to initiate antidepressant medication after determining that depressive symptoms are present. In the managed care environment, medical providers feel great pressure to initiate treatment rapidly, and it takes forbearance to temporize, to wait. Our point of view is that when alcohol-induced depression is suspected, it is wise to refrain from prescribing antidepressants for at least a week or more after the end of the drinking bout, and preferably for up to three weeks (Atkinson, 1999).

If antidepressants are given immediately, and the depression subsequently resolves, what does this prove? We know that alcohol-induced depression is much more prevalent than true comorbid depression, and that alcohol-induced depression resolves spontaneously: such depression gets better with or without medication. Therefore, if the improvement is attributed to the medication, this attribution will be false much more often than it will be true, and the parallel conclusion that a comorbid depression existed will also be false. Well, so what? you may ask. What harm has been done? We think several problems can arise from this false attribution. For one thing, it may very well lead to longer-term maintenance treatment with the antidepressant, which is costly, potentially hazardous, and, in a clientele noted for unreliable use of psychoactive substances in general, may be misused or perhaps shared with others. Moreover, a false diagnosis of a comorbid depressive disorder can become entrenched in the medical record and influence future (mis)diagnosis and treatment. Such consequences are in fact commonplace in large health care organizations.

On the other hand, depression should be treated early when the history suggests a comorbid disorder, e.g., a history of prior depressive episodes during abstinent periods, strong positive family history of depression, when there is no sign of even slight improvement in the first 7 to 14 days, or when strong suicidal intent persists after the first few days. Everyone would agree that syndromal depression persisting beyond 3 to 4 weeks' sobriety constitutes a true comorbid depression requiring vigorous antidepressant treatment (Brown et al., 1995). Several studies have shown that treatment of concurrent comorbid depression not only benefits depression but also improves drinking outcomes in younger alcoholics (reviewed in Atkinson, 1999). There is no reason to assume it should be otherwise in older patients.

Treating Depression in Patients Who Continue to Drink

What should clinicians do for depressed alcoholic outpatients who continue to drink despite efforts to dissuade them? Many such patients do not acknowledge the severity of their drinking behavior or refuse to participate in an alcoholism treatment program, yet they do want help for their depressive symptoms. Often, as in case 3 above, it may not be clear to what extent continuing depression is alcohol induced. One easily justified view is that such patients should not be treated with antidepressants until they stop drinking. This view was especially well founded in the past, because serious toxic effects of the early classes of available antidepressants, such as the tricyclic and heterocyclic drugs, were increased by alcohol excess. Thus orthostatic hypotension, cardiac arrhythmias, hepatotoxicity, and seizures were more likely to occur in patients taking these compounds who also drank heavily. Newer drugs, such as the selective serotonin reuptake inhibitors (SSRIs), produce less hazardous toxic reactions, so that the health risks of drinking while taking these medications are somewhat less worrisome. Nevertheless it is prudent to recognize that the majority of active heavy drinkers with depressive symptoms are likely to have some degree of alcohol-induced depression, and that in these cases prescribing an antidepressant medication does not fully address the cause of the depressive symptoms.

The decision to prescribe the newer antidepressants to a patient who continues to drink should be made on a case-by-case basis, weighing several factors listed below (see also Table 4.1). The more such factors appear to apply in a given case, the greater the justification for moving ahead with antidepressant treatment, even in the face of continued drinking.

1) *Severity of depression*: When suicidal intent or other severe depressive symptoms significantly impair functional status and endanger the patient's well-being, and symptom severity does not improve after the patient is no longer acutely intoxicated, treatment with medication for depression may be indicated (Cornelius et al., 1995). Often in such circumstances, the patient is hospitalized and treatment can at least be initiated in the sober state. A recent multisite study reported on alcohol consumption in 2,200 patients age 60 and older who required hospitalization for the management of depression at one of 71 geriatric psychiatry inpatient units (Oslin, Katz, Edell, & Ten Have, 2000). Eleven percent were consuming alcohol in the six months before admission. Most were light, presumably "social" drinkers; just 3.5% were daily drinkers. A large subsample of over 1,000 of these patients were then followed up, three to four months after hospital discharge. Among this group, over 80% of those patients who had been drinking before admission had reduced their alcohol use by more than 90% from preadmission levels. While it is likely that many patients were advised to reduce or stop drinking, because this is customary when patients are treated with antidepressant medications to reduce alcohol-drug interaction hazards, we have no assurance that this was done systematically. Yet even the heaviest daily drinkers, many of whom would probably have qualified for the diagnosis of an alcohol use disorder, had substantially reduced their intake. With regard to depression and functional status, these drinkers fared as well as nondrinkers at followup.

2) *Evidence for true comorbidity*: Were depressive symptoms present prior to the onset of an alcohol use disorder or during long abstinent intervals? This can be difficult to ascertain in older patients, many of whom began drinking in young adulthood. Collateral information from relatives may help. If the history clearly indicates prior depressive symptoms independent of drinking, antidepressant treatment may be warrant-

ed despite continuing use of alcohol. One placebo-controlled study of actively drinking alcoholic patients (mixed ages) with comorbid depression showed that patients treated with imipramine, but not those treated with placebo, experienced improvement in depression and reduction in alcohol consumption (McGrath et al., 1996).

3) *Frailty*: A patient's overall functional status, determined by all concurrent medical problems and treatments, will necessarily influence the clinician's judgment about whether to prescribe an antidepressant: generally, the frailer the patient, the more cautious one should be.

4) *Family history of depression*: If there is a strong family history of depressive illness or suicide, it is more likely that the patient is suffering from a truly comorbid depression that would benefit from medication, even in the face of current alcohol use (Roy, 1996).

5) *Pattern of adherence in treatment*: Often outpatients who fail to comply with an expectation of reduced drinking or abstinence also have difficulty adhering to other aspects of treatment. They may fail to attend scheduled appointments or report taking other medications erratically. If, on the other hand, a patient has been reliable in attending scheduled visits and adherent with other aspects of treatment, aside from being able to refrain from alcohol use, one may be justified in initiating antidepressant medication.

6) *Caregiver availability*: Supportive family, friends, or other caregivers may be enlisted to help assure reliable use of prescribed antidepressants. In the absence of such caregivers, greater caution is needed in prescribing.

Cognitive Deficits and Dementia

Among alcoholics, cognitive impairment related to excessive drinking increases with age, especially after age 50 (this subject is reviewed in detail in Atkinson, 2000). While alcoholics of any age are likely to experience transient difficulties with memory and attention after prolonged heavy drinking, in older patients these reversible deficits are not only more severe but take longer to resolve, showing incremental improvement that in some cases continues for months or even years after the last drink. When such cognitive impairment is minimal or transient—lasting no more than a week or two—one typically does not diagnose a separate disorder, but when cognitive loss persists, even if slowly improving, a comorbid diagnosis is required to indicate the persistent subsyndromal cognitive loss, e.g., "cognitive disorder not otherwise specified" with an added phrase that this is alcohol induced (American Psychiatric Association, 1994). In one well-evaluated case series, 19% of hospitalized alcoholics age 65 and older also suffered from such deficits (Finlayson, Hurt, Davis Jr., & Morse, 1988). The next case provides an example of severe but reversible cognitive loss:

Case 4: Alcohol Dependence With Slowly Resolving Cognitive Impairment and Alcohol-Induced Depression and Psychosis. RO, a 73-year-old divorced, unemployed man, was admitted to a general psychiatric ward because of suicidal thoughts and auditory hallucinations. He was acutely intoxicated with alcohol at the time of admission. He had drunk alcohol heavily for 30 to 40 years, without a significant abstinent period. At admission he also had significant cognitive and functional deficits. He was not able to manage his personal finances, and as a result his sister had been appointed as his legal conservator. In the hospital, antidepressant and antipsychotic medications were prescribed and his depressive and psychotic symptoms improved. However, significant residual cognitive and functional deficits required that he be placed in an assisted living facility after discharge. He was also referred to an outpatient alcoholism treatment program, but he failed to follow through.

Less than a year later, he left the facility and resumed independent living although his family opposed this. He stopped his medications and relapsed on alcohol soon thereafter. He was readmitted to the psychiatric ward, again acutely intoxicated, suicidal, and hearing voices. Medications were resumed and he was soon discharged back to the same assisted living facility he had left previously. In the following year two more psychiatric hospital admissions were necessary, each associated with drinking relapses, despite his continuing to reside in the supervised facility. Cognitive testing at the last admission included a score of 18/30 on the MMSE, consistent with mild to moderate dementia.

After this last hospital episode, and for the next two years, outpatient mental health staff worked more closely with him and he became successfully engaged in an outpatient group alcoholism treatment program for older adults. He remained abstinent during this time and did not exhibit any depressive or psychotic symptoms. His psychiatrist was able to taper and later discontinue all medications without difficulty or relapse. In addition, he showed gradual improvement in functional and cognitive performance. These changes were clinically noticeable after a few months of sustained sobriety, and after one and one half years of sobriety his MMSE score had improved to 25/30, in the low normal range. In the past three months, with the support of the treatment staff, he has returned to independent living and has legally regained control of his finances. He continues to remain abstinent and engaged in his alcoholism treatment program. He tells the staff these days that he "feels like a new person."

Case Discussion. This case touches on a number of important issues, beginning with the effects of long-term heavy drinking on cognitive performance and associated functional disabilities. Especially in older adults, it may require an extended interval of sobriety before full resolution of cognitive impairment occurs. In the cognitively impaired older alcoholic in treatment, frequent reassessment of cognitive status and provision by treatment staff of necessary support to regain functional capacities following improvement are important parts of the treatment plan (in this case, restored cognitive function made it possible for the patient to reestablish independent living and management of his finances).

This case also demonstrates the acute effects of heavy alcohol use on perception as well as on mood. The presence of depressive and psychotic symptoms with alcohol use, and subsequent lack of such symptoms during an extended period of sobriety, supports the diagnoses of alcohol-induced depressive and psychotic disorders. This patient's complex psychiatric situation also shows that multiple comorbid disorders can co-occur in the aging alcoholic. Finally, this case also dramatically illustrates the rewards of persistent professional efforts over the long term to pursue rehabilitation in the case of a complex, chronically alcoholic older adult.

Heavy drinking in persons with longstanding alcohol dependence can also cause a full-blown dementia that may be permanent (Atkinson, 2000; Oslin, Atkinson, Smith & Hendrie, 1998; Smith & Atkinson, 1995). Alcohol-induced persisting dementias account for 20% to 25% of cases in dementia registries, and have been diagnosed in 12% to 25% of older alcoholics in treatment (Atkinson, Ryan & Turner, 2000a; Finlayson et al., 1988). Here is an example:

Case 5: Alcohol Dependence With Probable Comorbid Alcohol-Induced Persisting Dementia. EB, a 77-year-old retired cook, was admitted to the medical ward following an alcohol withdrawal seizure that occurred shortly after he entered a local detoxification center where he was well known. He had consumed alcohol to the point of intoxication nearly every day for the past 50 years, had had multiple arrests for drunken driving and public intoxication, and in recent years lived in a single room occupancy hotel in a poor section of the inner city. Recently he had been drinking a pint to a fifth of whiskey daily.

When admitted to the ward he was drowsy but rousable, disoriented except to person, and unable to participate in other cognitive testing. Extraocular eye movements were intact, and there was no nystagmus or gaze preference. His blood alcohol level was still 125 mg/100 ml. A CT scan of the brain showed generalized atrophy of the cerebral cortex and cerebellum. A week after entering the hospital, following uneventful withdrawal from alcohol and doses of intramuscular thiamine, he scored 18/30 on the MMSE, well within the range for a presumptive diagnosis of dementia, with deficits in attention, orientation, and memory.

Cognitive deficits improved somewhat but still persisted during the patient's subsequent 9-month stay in a closed, alcohol-free nursing home. He was then referred to the dementia clinic, where his MMSE score as 21/30. Performance on other neuropsychological tests showed marked impairment of attention, short-term memory, similarities and visual-constructional skills, but only mild impairment in language repetition, judgment, and calculation. Language comprehension and naming ability were intact. Neurological examination showed marked impairment of tandem gait and a positive Romberg test. There was symmetrical bilateral loss of proprioception and vibratory sensation in his feet.

Case Discussion. This man's situation illustrates findings commonly seen in cases where alcohol appears to be a major factor in dementia: namely, a history of prolonged, heavy alcohol consumption; persistent, widespread cognitive impairment with sparing of naming ability; associated neurological findings of peripheral polyneuropathy and ataxia; brain imaging evidence of diffuse cortical and cerebellar atrophy; and no evidence of further cognitive decline (a stable course or perhaps even slight improvement) with abstention from alcohol.

Faced with an older alcoholic patient who suffers from comorbid dementia, the clinician must attempt to determine whether the dementia is related to the alcohol use disorder or instead represents the more common disorder of Alzheimer's dementia, or another type of dementia. Accurate dementia diagnosis has important prognostic significance for the patient and family: alcohol-induced persisting dementia may plateau or improve with abstinence, but Alzheimer's and other degenerative dementias will worsen over time. The distinction in diagnosis is not always easy, is not well delineated by current DSM-IV criteria, and may require repeated observation and testing over time. Table 4.2 lists some potentially useful criteria for distinguishing between Alzheimer's and alcohol-related dementia.

Table 4.2 Alcohol-Related Versus Alzheimer's Dementia[a]

Feature	Alcohol-Induced Persisting Dementia	Alzheimer's Dementia
Meets criteria for dementia	+	+
Cortical atrophy on MRI	+	+
Long history of heavy drinking	+	–
Ataxia may be present	+	–
Peripheral polyneuropathy may be present	+	–
Cerebellar atrophy may be present on MRI	+	–
Abstinence halts cognitive decline	+	–
Cortical atrophy can be reversed	+	–
Anomia/dysnomia prominent	–	+
Cognitive decline continues despite abstinence	–	+
CSF "tau" protein may be elevated	–	+

Note. Based on Morikawa et al., 1999; Oslin et al., 1998; Smith & Atkinson, 1995. Adapted with permission.

[a]Symbols "+" and "–" mean that the finding is more (+) or less (–) likely to be associated with this form of dementia; MRI = magnetic resonance imaging of the brain; CSF = cerebrospinal fluid.

Treatment and Management

Irrespective of the cause of dementia, patients with mild to moderate cognitive impairment may still be productively engaged in an alcohol treatment program, provided that the methods of treatment are tailored to their capacities. A slow pace and emotional support are essential. It is important to organize information into small, concrete units, and to repeat a unit of information until staff are certain, through solicited feedback or paraphrasing by the client, that the material has been understood. Cognitive-behavioral methods are especially useful because they characteristically employ such techniques. For patients with more severe or worsening dementias, treatment in alcoholism treatment programs is not likely to be productive and, in group-based programs, can hamper the treatment of others. Nevertheless, it is important to abate alcohol use in anyone suffering from Alzheimer's or any other dementia, because continued drinking in the face of dementia hastens cognitive decline (Teri, Hughes & Larson, 1990) and is associated with high rates of early mortality (Simon, Epstein & Reynolds, 1968). Day care, foster home care, and residential and assisted living programs are among the options to be considered in these cases. When demented patients continue to drink even after placements in such settings as these, a closed, alcohol-free residential setting may be necessary (case 5).

Anxiety

Alcohol withdrawal can induce anxiety symptoms in almost anyone. If a social drinker imbibes several drinks and thus establishes a significant blood alcohol level, as that level declines in the ensuing hours after the last drink there will be a tendency for the individual to experience some degree of autonomic nervous system arousal—perhaps some sweating, heart palpitations, awakening from sleep or restlessness—and, not uncommonly, subjective nervous tension or mild anxiety. This represents alcohol withdrawal-induced anxiety and usually lasts for just an hour or two in non-alcoholic drinkers. Alcoholic drinkers, even if they do not suffer from a true comorbid anxiety disorder, may experience more frequent and distressing alcohol-withdrawal anxiety because their customary drinking through the day and evening leads to continual ups and downs in alcohol blood level.

Persons who are heavily dependent on alcohol may suffer extremely unpleasant anxiety symptoms during alcohol withdrawal, without delirium, and this is properly diagnosed as alcohol-induced anxiety. These acute and distressing symptoms should of course be treated with a brief regimen of anxiolytic, sedative medication, usually benzodiazepines, but the need for such drugs to cover withdrawal anxiety should be concluded within a week or less. When anxiety symptoms persist beyond the usual time course for resolution of alcohol withdrawal, these symptoms may signal the presence of a comorbid anxiety disorder.

Whether there is more than a coincidental association between alcohol use disorders and true comorbid anxiety disorders is at this time a matter of controversy: there is published evidence from studies of younger alcoholics that both supports (e.g., Kushner, Sher, & Erickson, 1999) and fails to support (e.g., Schuckit & Hesselbrock, 1994) the idea that anxiety disorders are more common in alcoholics than in the general population. In case series of older alcoholics, anxiety disorders are certainly common enough, coexisting in 4% to 26% of patients, although these disorders tend to be less commonly reported than depression and cognitive problems. Persons with these disorders are difficult to epitomize, because this diagnostic group is so heterogeneous: generalized anxiety, panic, phobic, obsessive-compulsive, and post-traumatic stress disorders are all in this group. Unlike the depressive disorders, in which similar symptoms characterize them all, the cardinal symptoms of each type of anxiety disorder differ from the others. It is our experience that in some patients, longstanding phobic, generalized anxiety or mild obsessive-compulsive symptoms may be overshadowed by symptoms of more acute and emotionally painful depression and worry about life stressors, and thus may be overlooked.

As in depression, alcohol can be used as self-medication by alcoholic and reactive heavy drinkers to attenuate symptoms of nervous tension, anxiety, and irritability (Dupree & Schonfeld, 1998). A number of military combat veterans in our VA-based treatment program for older alcoholics—men who had experienced extremely traumatic events during WW II, the Korean Conflict, or the Vietnam War—complain that after achieving sobriety their PTSD symptoms, such as reexperiencing traumatic events in dreams or when awake, tend to become worse, possibly because they no longer use alcohol to suppress these symptoms. Because of the self-medication phenomenon, accurate diagnosis and treatment of anxiety disorders helps remove a risk factor for drinking relapses.

Treatment

Until recently the only available medications for these disorders were problematic, especially for older adults. Tricyclic antidepressants are very effective for panic disorder and some cases of PTSD, but their side effect profiles are unsatisfactory for many older adults (e.g., anticholinergic effects, orthostatic hypotension, cardiac conduction abnormalities). Benzodiazepines benefit patients with generalized anxiety disorders but when used over long periods carry risks, particularly in aging persons, for cumulative toxicity (daytime sedation, drowsiness, deficits in attention and memory), actual increases in anxiety and depression (possibly present in case 2), and physical dependence even on low doses. Dependence liability of benzodiazepines is greater among alcoholics. Fortunately, the newer antidepressants, especially the SSRIs, can in many cases offer effective control of symptoms in all varieties of anxiety disorders, with much safer side effect and toxicity profiles and virtually no dependence liability. Psychotherapy and behavioral treatments are often also necessary in more entrenched cases.

Comorbid Drug Use

The most common comorbid substance use disorder found among aging alcoholics is tobacco (nicotine) dependence—regular, daily cigarette smoking, which is an active problem in a strikingly high 50% to 70% of patients. This prevalence level is four to five times greater than smoking rates in the general aging population. Comorbid dependence upon prescription drugs—mainly anxiolytic and sedative-hypnotics of the benzodiazepine class and opioid analgesics—has been reported in up to 14% of hospitalized alcoholics age 65 and older (Finlayson et al., 1988). Reports of illicit drug use in this population vary, but most programs report evidence of only sporadic, subsyndromal use of cocaine, illicit opioids or marijuana. In our program, for example, about 5% of older alcoholic patients report such drug use. Typically older alcoholics are introduced to illicit drugs by younger relatives or sexual partners.

General Issues in Assessment and Treatment

Comorbid psychiatric disorders are so common in this population that assessment by a certified mental health professional should be a routine aspect of every initial comprehensive assessment. Programs need access to psychiatrists and psychologists for specialized diagnostic assessments and treatments when indicated. It is ideal when these specialists have integral liaison roles on the treatment team (Atkinson, Turner & Tolson, 1998). As suggested in our introductory comments, counselors and case managers who treat older alcoholics need to be grounded in basic principles of work with mentally ill patients. Programs that treat older clients with major comorbid mental disorders must be able to arrange timely psychiatric emergency evaluation and hospitalization when needed.

As already discussed, treatment of concurrent depression improves drinking outcomes of alcoholics comorbid for this mood disorder. The same can be said in principle for treatment of anxiety disorders, although evidence is lacking to show that improved drinking outcomes follow effective treatment of comorbid anxiety disorders.

Cigarette smoking poses far greater risks for morbidity and mortality than any other form of substance abuse. Every alcoholism treatment program should provide, or have ready access to, a smoking cessation program; effective cessation methods have been tailored for older smokers (see chapter 10 in this volume). Treatment of prescription drug dependence is considered elsewhere (Atkinson, 2000; chapter 9 in this volume). Perhaps we should also add that any elderly patient who is being treated with prescribed psychoactive medications for a mental disorder needs to be advised not to drink alcoholic beverages while taking such medications.

Does Psychiatric Comorbidity Compromise the Outcome of Alcoholism Treatment?

When adequate mental health assessment and treatment services are provided, comorbidity does *not* diminish the chances that older alcoholics will benefit from treatment of their drinking problems. In a recent study of 110 consecutive patients—60% of whom had comorbid psychiatric disorders—treated in an alcoholism program designed for older adults that offers "built in" geriatric psychiatry services, our group found that patients with comorbid disorders were as likely to complete a year of outpatient treatment as those without a comorbid condition (Atkinson et al., 1998; Atkinson, Ryan & Turner, 2000b). Blow's group found the same thing for 6-month drinking outcomes following age-specific inpatient alcoholism treatment: older patients with comorbid disorders fared as well as the others (Blow, Walton, Chermack, Mudd, & Brower, 2000). This is good news.

Acknowledgment

We thank Drs. Rob Olsen (case 2) and David M. Smith (case 5) for providing two of the case vignettes.

References

American Psychiatric Association. (1994). *Diagnostic and statistical manual of mental disorders,* (4th ed.). Washington, DC: Author.

Atkinson, R. M. (1998). The psychosocial impact of alcoholism in older adults: Consequences, complications and comorbidities. *The Southwest Journal on Aging, 14,* 73–83.

Atkinson, R. M. (1999). Depression, alcoholism and aging: A brief review. *International Journal of Geriatric Psychiatry, 14,* 905–910.

Atkinson, R. M. (2000). Substance abuse. In C. E. Coffee and J. L. Cummings (Editors), *Textbook of Geriatric Neuropsychiatry,* (2nd ed.), pp. 367–400. Washington, DC: American Psychiatric Press.

Atkinson, R. M., Ryan, S. C., & Turner, J. A. (2000 a). Variation among aging alcoholics in treatment (in preparation).

Atkinson, R. M., Ryan, S. C., & Turner, J. A. (2000 b). Predicting treatment adherence of older alcoholic men: Patient profiles and pathways into treatment (in preparation).

Atkinson, R. M., Turner, J. A., & Tolson, R. L. (1998). Treatment of older adult problem drinkers: Lessons learned from the "Class of '45." *Journal of Mental Health and Aging, 4,* 197–214.

Blow, F. C., Cook, C. A. L., Booth, B. M., Falcon, S. P., & Friedman, M. J. (1992). Age-related psychiatric comorbidities and level of functioning in alcoholic veterans seeking outpatient treatment. *Hospital and Community Psychiatry, 43,* 990–995.

Blow, F. C., Walton, M. A., Chermack, S. T., Mudd, S. A., & Brower, K. J. (2000). Older adult treatment outcome following elder-specific inpatient alcoholism treatment. *Journal of Substance Abuse Treatment* (in press).

Brown, S. A., & Schuckit, M. A. (1988). Changes in depression among abstinent alcoholics. *Journal of Studies on Alcohol, 49,* 412–417.

Brown, S. A., Inaba, R. K., Gillin, J. C., Schuckit, M. A., Stewart, M. A., & Irwin, M. R. (1995). Alcoholism and affective disorder: Clinical course of depressive symptoms. *American Journal of Psychiatry, 152,* 45–52.

Cornelius, J. R., Salloum, I. M., Mezzich, J., Cornelius, M. D., Fabrega, Jr. H., Ehler, J. G., Ulrich, R. F., Thase, M. E., & Mann, J. J. (1995). Disproportionate suicidality in patients with comorbid major depression and alcoholism. *American Journal of Psychiatry, 152,* 358–364.

Dupree, L. W., & Schonfeld, L. (1998). Cognitive-behavioral and self-management treatment of older problem drinkers. *Journal of Mental Health and Aging, 4,* 215–232.

Finlayson, R. E., Hurt, R. D., Davis, Jr., L. J., & Morse, R. M. (1988). Alcoholism in elderly persons: A study of the psychiatric and psychosocial features of 216 inpatients. *Mayo Clinic Proceedings, 63,* 761–768.

Kushner, M. G., Sher, K. J., & Erickson, D. J. (1999). Prospective analysis of the relation between DSM-III anxiety disorders and alcohol use disorders. *American Journal of Psychiatry, 156,* 723–732.

McGrath, P. J., Nunes, E. V., Stewart, J. W., Goldman, D., Agosti, V., Ocepek-Welikson, K., & Quitkin, F. M. (1996). Imipramine treatment of alcoholics with major depression: A placebo-controlled clinical trial. *Archives of General Psychiatry, 53,* 232–240.

Morikawa, Y-I, Arai, H., Matsushita, S., Kato, M., Higuchi, S., Miura, M., Kawakami, H., Higuchi, M., Okamura, N., Tashiro, M., Matsui, T., & Sasaki, H. (1999). Cerebrospinal fluid tau protein levels in demented and nondemented alcoholics. *Alcoholism: Clinical and Experimental Research, 23,* 575–577.

Morse, R. M., & Flavin, D. K. (1992). The definition of alcoholism. *Journal of the American Medical Association, 268,* 1012–1014.

Oslin, D., Atkinson, R. M., Smith, D. M., & Hendrie, H. (1998). Alcohol-related dementia: Proposed clinical criteria. *International Journal of Geriatric Psychiatry, 13,* 203–212.

Oslin, D. W., Katz, I. R., Edell, W. S., & Ten Have, T. R. (2000). Effects of alcohol consumption on the treatment of depression among elderly patients. *American Journal of Geriatric Psychiatry, 8,* 215–220.

Roy, A. (1996). Aetiology of secondary depression in male alcoholics. *British Journal of Psychiatry, 169,* 753–757.

Schuckit, M. A., & Hesselbrock, V. (1994). Alcohol dependence and anxiety disorders: What is the relationship? *American Journal of Psychiatry, 151,* 1723–1734.

Schutte, K. K., Brennan, P. L., & Moos, R. H. (1998). Predicting the development of late-life late-onset drinking problems: A 7–year prospective study. *Alcoholism: Clinical and Experimental Research, 22,* 1349–1358.

Simon, A., Epstein, L. J., & Reynolds, L. (1968). Alcoholism in the geriatric mentally ill. *Geriatrics, 23,* 125–131.

Smith, D. M., & Atkinson, R. M. (1995). Alcoholism and dementia. *International Journal of the Addictions, 30,* 1843–1869.

Teri, L., Hughes, J. P., & Larson, E. B. (1990). Cognitive deterioration in Alzheimer's Disease: Behavioral and health factors. *Journal of Gerontology, 45,* 58–63.

5

Alcoholism, Drug Abuse, and Suicide in the Elderly

George E. Murphy

Suicide is nearly always a consequence of psychiatric illness. Only a very few suicides are found to have been without such affliction (Cheng, 1995; Rich, Young, & Fowler, 1986; Robins, Murphy, Wilkinson, Gassner, & Kayes, 1959). Major depressive disorder accounts for roughly half of the total. Alcoholism and other substance abuse together comprise the second largest contributor to suicide. They are found in 25%–40% of self-inflicted deaths annually (Robins et al., 1959). When not the primary diagnosis, major depressive disorder is yet found to have complicated the clinical picture in about two-thirds of the substance abusers (Murphy, Wetzel, Robins, & McEvoy, 1992), so depression must be regarded as the leading player in suicide.

Only in the last 10 years has any serious attention been paid to suicide in the elderly. It is known that the suicide rate in men (given as the number of such deaths per 100,000 live population of like age and sex) rises steeply and steadily, beginning at age 65 years. The corresponding rate in women, only one-fourth that of men overall, starts a slow decline at about the same age. Meanwhile, the proportion of suicides attributable to substance abuse declines as well in both sexes, replaced by greater numbers suffering with major depression (Carney, Rich, Burke, & Fowler, et al., 1994; Conwell et al., 1996).

The last 30 years or so have seen a steady and dismaying rise in the illicit use of narcotic and stimulant drugs among the young. As an antecedent to suicide, such drug abuse has, to a large extent, replaced alcoholism as the second most common psychiatric diagnosis in the under-30 age group (Rich, Fowler, Fogarty, & Young, 1988). Abuse of illicit drugs appears to decline sharply by middle age and is only rarely represented among suicides in the later years of life. Among prescription sedatives, the barbiturates have been replaced in the medical armamentarium by the much safer benzodiazepines, e.g. Librium®, Valium®, Ativan®, and Xanax®. These anxiolytics, now widely prescribed, are inefficient as agents of suicide. However, they all have the potential for abuse and addiction, with consequent negative social consequences, including suicide (Rich et al., 1988).

The original occasion for the anxiolytic prescription is commonly a personal crisis of one sort or another with attendant depression. Anxiety or insomnia or both may be the most striking complaints. All too often, the family physician treats the symptom but fails to search for the underlying mood disorder (Murphy, 1975; Oquendo, Malone, Ellis, Sacheim, & Mann, 1999). Untreated, it worsens, and so does the insomnia. Larger or more frequent doses of sedative are requested, reinforcing the focus on the symptom. If the physician becomes uneasy about the escalating dosage and attempts to cut it back, a dramatic outbreak of complaints threatens the doctor-patient relationship and he/she may feel trapped into continuing to overprescribe.

Abusers of one substance are at increased risk of abusing another, and it doesn't seem to matter which comes first. An example of this progression is the following:

> Helen had married at 19. She sought no advancement beyond high school, but she worked to help her husband earn his college degree and a master's in business administration. Thereafter, she no longer worked outside of the home. When her mother became senile, she went to live with her. Under that strain and her husband's frequent business trips Helen developed a depression with marked insomnia. Her family physician treated the symptom with barbiturate hypnotics and missed the depression. She abused the sedative for relief of symptoms and for relief from problems of her unsatisfying existence. Because of her frequent drug intoxication, the emotional gap between her husband and herself widened. Soon, they occupied separate bedrooms. She abandoned the friends she had formerly enjoyed, preferring to escape into oblivion. When her mother died, Helen was consumed with guilt and developed more florid symptoms of depression. She began to augment her sedative medication with alcohol and became alcohol dependent as well. She

spoke of suicide on a number of occasions. A very serious suicide attempt by overdose of hypnotic medication while her husband was away was thwarted by the unexpected arrival of relatives. She was uncooperative with psychiatric treatment and did not benefit. She hated the periodic hospitalizations occasioned by her aggressive outbursts when intoxicated. Finally, under threat of involuntary commitment, she took an overdose of a hypnotic drug, washed down with alcohol, and died at the age of 60.

The Progression to Suicide

The progression to suicide is similar in alcoholism and other substance abuse but different in affective disorder (Duberstein, Conwell, & Caine, 1993; Murphy & Robins, 1967; Rich et al., 1988). In the latter, little disturbance in the external aspects of life is seen (Murphy & Robins, 1967). For example, depressives who take their lives usually have what appears to be a good social support system. Their economic status is less often a problem compared with substance abusers (Murphy & Robins, 1967). They do tend to have substantially poorer health than nonsuicides of like age (Rich et al., 1988), but other stressors are not found to be greater in number or severity than is to be expected in the general population. The impetus to suicide is internally or psychologically driven. Joylessness, misery, and especially hopelessness seem to be the motivation (Beck, Brown, Berchick, Stewart, & Steer, 1990). When one observes the depth and impenetrability of the hopelessness that may develop, one can more easily understand choosing death.

Substance abusers, in contrast to pure depressives, react strongly to external events, particularly to loss of a close interpersonal relationship. Although originally observed in alcoholics (Murphy & Robins, 1967), this selectivity has been shown to be true regardless of the substance abused (Rich et al., 1988). Marital separation, divorce, breakup of a dependent or love relationship, estrangement, bereavement, all have contributed to suicide in substance abusers. Much of this disruption is a consequence of the substance abuser's own behavior. Chaotic and disrupted relationships are a common part of their experience. Half of a group of 34 alcoholics had experienced at least one disruption in the year preceding their suicide (Murphy & Robins, 1967). The same was found to be true in a further series of 50 alcoholic suicides (Murphy, Armstrong, Hermele, Fischer, & Clendenin, 1979). But in both series nearly two-thirds of these events had occurred *within the last six weeks of their lives.* Similar findings are reported by Rich et al. (1988) and by Duberstein et al. (1993). The distribution of these events is clearly skewed, and is irrespective of age. What, then, gave these events their lethal potency? In all cases but one, the disrupted relationship, however ambivalently regarded, was the last meaningful one in that person's world. This is illustrated in the following vignette.

> Robert was an easygoing and cheerful man who married a domineering and abusive woman before he was old enough to know better. He was a good worker and well liked, but a binge drinker who had been arrested many times for drunkenness and peace disturbance. When his wife began to see another man, some three years before his death, he became sad, cried easily, and lost interest in socializing. His drinking increased, and he had trouble maintaining employment. When he could no longer hold a job, she refused to give him money and repeatedly humiliated him. He spoke of suicide on a number of occasions and asked his brother to pay for his funeral. His wife threw him out of the house a month before his suicide. He then lived in transient quarters where he hanged himself with a bedsheet thrown over the transom. He was 63 years old.

In the absence of interpersonal loss, other calamities have befallen, or are about to befall the substance abuser who takes his/her own life. Being jailed or facing imprisonment is one such final straw. Facing disfiguring surgery, severe financial reversal, marked loss of status, or humiliation can precipitate a suicide as well (Murphy, 1992). But loss of the last emotional support seems to be the most potent precipitant, as illustrated by Teddy's case.

> Teddy was 61, a lifelong bachelor. He had always lived with his mother, and they were emotionally dependent on each other. She made all of the family decisions. She and her husband, Teddy's father, had gone their separate ways years earlier. Although regularly employed, Teddy drank daily, often to excess. Because his mother would not allow alcohol in the house, he often drank and slept in his car in the garage. He dated women, and would stay with one or another of them when on a bender. Eight months before his suicide, Teddy's mother was diagnosed with pelvic cancer, and both of them were distraught. He gradually became depressed with insomnia, loss of appetite, interest and energy, and talked of suicide. He saw a physician about his "nerves." The doctor recognized the depression but prescribed only a popular sedative for his insomnia. When his mother's condition required her

> terminal hospitalization, his depression worsened. He quit work, drank less and less, and was underactive. A week before his death, he quarreled with his girlfriend and she refused to see him again. He shot himself in the garage. His mother lived only a week longer. All of his support system was gone.

Vigorous treatment of the depression might have changed the outcome for him, but he did not know how to live his own life.

Suicide is a late complication of substance abuse. Among alcoholics the mean duration from onset of alcohol abuse to suicide is about 20 years, but the older the age of onset the shorter that interval becomes (Murphy, 1992). More often than not, a depressive episode supervenes, engrafted upon the substance abuse. The disorders are then said to be *comorbid.* (See chapter 4 in this volume.) Depression carries its own risk of suicide as mentioned previously. The combination may be all it takes to tip the scales to self-destruction.

Estimating the Risk of Suicide

While these loss events may help us understand the suicidal decision in aging substance abusers, what is needed is a way of estimating risk in advance of the dire event. Seven markers, none of them lethal, appear to be additive in their impact (Murphy et al., 1992) (see Table 5.1). In a large series of alcohol suicides, 90% had at least three of the seven markers: 82% had four or more. This has been demonstrated to be very different from the circumstances in living alcoholics (Murphy et al., 1992). Attention to these markers makes it possible to monitor the worsening or lessening of suicide risk in the individual patient. Add to these the well-established risk that a family history of suicide or suicide attempts entails.

Table 5.1 Additional Risk Factors for Suicide in Substance Abusers

1. Continued substance abuse
2. Expressed suicidal thoughts/attempt
3. Little social support
4. Concurrent depression
5. Poor physical health
6. Loss/lack of employment
7. Living alone

Preventing Suicide

The cornerstone of suicide prevention is the successful recognition and treatment of the underlying psychiatric illness. The first step is diagnosis. Both depression and substance use disorders are frequently found to have been undiagnosed, underdiagnosed, or undertreated before suicide (Isacsson, Boëthius, & Bergman, 1992; Murphy, 1975). Physicians too frequently prescribe anxiolytic (sedative) medication instead of adequate antidepressant treatment, and thereby lose the opportunity to quickly relieve a potentially lethal depression (Isaccson et al., 1992; Murphy, 1975). The potentially disastrous consequence of a missed diagnosis emphasizes the need to be alert to both diagnoses.

A comprehensive effort in a region of Denmark to acquaint or reacquaint all family practice physicians with the diagnosis and treatment of major depression resulted in a statistically significant reduction in the number of suicides in the following year (Rutz, vonKnorring, & Wälinder, 1989). Subsequent analysis showed that "at the maximum effect of the programme, there was no suicide in the area by anyone treated solely by a general practitioner." (Rutz, vonKnorring, Pihlgren, Rihmer, & Wälinder, 1995) "[T]he 60% decrease of suicides after the programme was almost totally a result of a decrease in female suicides. The number of male suicides was almost unchanged." This illustrates that the difficulty both in getting men into treatment and in securing their cooperation (Murphy, 1998) is not confined to the United States. Nevertheless, it is clear that the suicides that occur under a physician's care are those that have fallen through the diagnostic/therapeutic net (Isacsson et al., 1992; Murphy, 1975).

A higher sensitivity to the variety of presentations of depression is needed. In the nonpsychiatric physician's practice, it often comes embedded in another disorder. Not the least of these is substance abuse. While maximum protection from suicide in substance abusers is achieved through abstinence, this is not readily accomplished. The comorbid diagnosis—major depression—is the critical element in a majority of cases. It is more easily treated than is the substance abuse, but first it must be recognized and vigorously treated.

Next, the level of suicide risk must be assessed. Suicide rating scales offer no improvement in detection over direct inquiry. It is essential to ask the patient or client directly about suicidal thoughts and acts, first on a "have you ever?" basis, then in the present. Have no fear that these questions will either introduce the idea or launch it into action. Alcoholics readily communicate such thoughts often intermittently for months or even years (Murphy et al., 1992). Both the intensity and frequency of these thoughts are relevant. One must monitor the waxing and waning of suicidal ideation. The subacute and chronic risk factors listed above come into play as a measure of risk. From a baseline of data obtained at first contact, monitor also the patient's social, vocational, and health changes. Assess the strength of social support and its changes, as this is often the area of greatest vulnerability.

Commonsense measures too often overlooked in the treatment of substance abusers are: (1) ask family members to report depressive symptoms and suicidal communications; (2) instruct family to *remove all firearms from the premises* (i.e., attempting to hide them at home is worse than useless); (3) brief hospitalization may help the patient over a suicidal crisis; (4) work to improve social connections.

Diagnosing Major Depressive Disorder

The diagnosis of depression is made in the same way as are other diagnoses in medical practice—by identifying the presence of a *syndrome.* This is a group of symptoms occurring simultaneously that together constitute the key feature of the diagnosis. Time can be saved at the outset by prescreening. The Beck Depression Inventory (BDI)©* is a self-report form a patient or client can be asked to fill out at the time of registration (Beck, Ward, Mendelson, Mock, & Erbaugh, 1961). It consists of 23 multiple choice statements regarding a range of depressive symptoms and is scored additively. A score of 10 or greater usually corresponds to significant depression.

Some investigators prefer to use the Geriatric Depression Scale (Yesavage, Brink, Rose, & Adey, 1983) in elderly patients. It is a self-report instrument that focuses entirely on thoughts and feelings. Both scales are assessments of severity, and are useful in monitoring change in intensity of depression. Neither is a diagnostic instrument. There is simply no substitute for a carefully conducted personal interview to establish a diagnosis of major depression. Thoughts, feelings, and physiological

*Copies available from: Psychological Corporation, 555 Academic Court, San Antonio, TX 78204–2498.

functioning (e.g., energy, sleep, appetite, concentration) are all part of the diagnosis.

Foremost is a disturbance of mood. Depressed individuals may report feeling sad, rather than depressed. Feeling blue, "down in the dumps," or "blah" are other ways of describing a depressed mood. The symptom has persisted for weeks if not longer. Anhedonia—inability to find pleasure in anything—is the alternative first criterion for the diagnosis. Disturbance in sleep pattern—persistent insomnia or hypersomnia—accompanies it. Loss of appetite (and often weight as well), loss of energy, interest, and concentration are diagnostic symptoms. Pronounced feelings of guilt or worthlessness, agitation or retardation (slowed thoughts and motion), and thoughts of death and/or of suicide complete the list of key symptoms. (See *Diagnostic and Statistical Manual of Mental Disorders,* 4th ed., American Psychiatric Association, 1994). *Any four of these, plus mood disturbance or pervasive loss of ability to enjoy, occurring together in time, identify the syndrome and diagnosis of depression.* The patient will not necessarily complain of these symptoms spontaneously, but will nearly always acknowledge their presence if asked—so ask. It is important to resist the tendency to discount a symptom, or the disorder itself, because it can be—or appears to be—linked to an identifiable stressor such as a loss or a physical illness. Inadequate or no treatment will be the result. "The presence of a 'reason' for depression does not constitute a good reason for ignoring its presence" (Fawcett, 1972). Recognition and vigorous treatment of depression can not only reduce the death toll, but much human suffering as well.

Treating Depression

Antidepressant pharmacotherapy, except in extreme cases, is the treatment of choice. The older antidepressants, most of them of a tricyclic chemical configuration, while effective, are highly toxic in overdose. The newer drugs, most notably the selective serotonin reuptake inhibitors, or SSRIs, are not. Thus, these newer drugs are best to use with often unreliable and impulsive substance abusers. With any antidepressant, it is essential to give a high enough dosage and for long enough. That means four to six weeks as a therapeutic trial (Donovan, Quitkin, & Stewart, 1994). When found, the effective drug should be administered continuously well beyond symptomatic improvement. Nonpsychiatrist physicians are commonly reluctant to prescribe an adequate daily dose. The low side-effect profile of the newer antidepressants makes this difficult to understand. Two psychotherapies, cognitive therapy and interpersonal therapy, have also been shown to have substantial efficacy in the treatment of mild to moderate depression. However, unless one is trained and skilled in their use, pharmacotherapy is the better choice.

Summary

Abuse of alcohol and of prescription medication is not rare beyond age 50. Complicating depression heightens suicide risk. Treating symptoms instead of the underlying disorders is the usual error in suicides occurring under medical care (Murphy, 1975). There is little danger of overdiagnosing major depression. It is very common in clinical practice. It is often the impetus for seeking consultation, although it may not be the chief complaint. Not every depression is a suicidal one, but all produce misery. Achieving the relief from that misery is imperative, and not difficult to accomplish—but first comes diagnosis. Direct inquiry regarding suicidal thoughts is necessary. There is no danger that it will plant or reinforce an idea.

Substance abusers are uniquely vulnerable to loss—of employment, health, status, but particularly of physical and emotional support. Acute changes in any of these call for careful assessment and whatever support can be mustered.

References

American Psychiatric Association. (1994). *Diagnostic and statistical manual of mental disorders* (4th ed.). Washington, DC: Author.

Beck, A. T., Brown, G., Berchick, R. J., Stewart, B. L., & Steer, R. A. (1990). Relationship between hopelessness and ultimate suicide: A replication with psychiatric outpatients. *American Journal of Psychiatry, 147,* 190–195.

Beck, A. T., Ward, C. H., Mendelson, M., Mock, J., & Erbaugh, J. (1961). An inventory for measuring depression. *Archives of General Psychiatry, 4,* 561–571.

Carney, S. S., Rich, C. L., Burke, P. A., & Fowler, R. C. (1994). Suicide over

60: The San Diego Study. *Journal of the American Geriatric Society, 42,* 174–180.

Cheng, A. T. A. (1995). Mental illness and suicide: A case-control study in East Taiwan. *Archives of General Psychiatry, 52,* 594–603.

Conwell, Y., Duberstein, P. R., Cox, C., Herrmann, J. H., Forbes, N. T., & Caine, E. D. (1996). Relationships of age and Axis I diagnoses in victims of completed suicide: A psychological autopsy study. *American Journal of Psychiatry, 153,* 1001–1008.

Donovan, S. J., Quitkin, F. M., & Stewart, J. S. (1994). Duration of antidepressant trials: Clinical and research implication. *Journal of Clinical Psychopharmacology, 14,* 64–66.

Duberstein, P. R., Conwell, Y., & Caine, E. D. (1993). Interpersonal stressors, substance abuse and suicide. *Journal of Nervous and Mental Disease, 181,* 80–85.

Fawcett, J. (1972). Suicidal depression and physical illness. *Journal of the American Medical Association, 219,* 1303–1306.

Isacsson, G., Boëthius, G., & Bergmann, V. (1992). Low-level of antidepressant prescription for people who later commit suicide: 15 years of experience from a population-based drug database in Sweden. *Acta Psychiatrica Scandinavica, 85,* 444–448.

Murphy, G. E. (1975). The physician's responsibility for suicide. II. Errors of omission. *Annals of Internal Medicine, 82,* 305–309.

Murphy, G. E. (1992). *Suicide in alcoholism.* New York: Oxford University Press.

Murphy, G. E. (1998). Why women are less likely than men to commit suicide. *Comprehensive Psychiatry, 39,* 1–12.

Murphy, G. E., Armstrong, J. W., Hermele, S. L., Fischer, J. R., & Clendenin, W. W. (1979). Suicide and alcoholism. Interpersonal loss confirmed as a predictor. *Archives of General Psychiatry, 36,* 65–69.

Murphy, G. E., & Robins, E. (1967). Social factors in suicide. *Journal of the American Medical Association, 199,* 303–308.

Murphy, G. E., Wetzel, R. D., Robins, E., & McEvoy, L, 1992. Multiple risk factors predict suicide in alcoholism. *Archives of General Psychiatry, 49,* 459–463.

Oquendo, M. A., Malone, K. M., Ellis, S. P., Sacheim, H. A., & Mann, J. J. (1999). Inadequacy of antidepressant treatment for patients with major depression who are at risk for suicidal behavior. *American Journal of Psychiatry, 156,* 190–194.

Rich, C. L., Fowler, R. C., Fogarty, L. A., & Young, D. (1988). San Diego suicide study: III. Relationships between diagnoses and stressors. *Archives of General Psychiatry, 45*, 589–592.

Rich, C. L., Young, D., & Fowler, R. C. (1986). San Diego suicide study: I. Young versus old subjects. *Archives of General Psychiatry, 43,* 577–582.

Robins, E., Murphy, G. E., Wilkinson, R. H., Gassner, S., & Kayes, J. (1959). Some clinical considerations in the prevention of suicide based on a study of 134 successful suicides. *American Journal of Public Health, 49,* 888–899.

Rutz, W., vonKnorring, L., & Wälinder, J. (1989). Frequency of suicide on Gotland after systematic postgraduate education of general practitioners. *Acta Psychiatrica Scandinavica, 80,* 151–154.

Rutz, W., vonKnorring, L., Pihlgren, H., Rihmer, Z., & Wälinder, J. (1995). Prevention of male suicides: Lessons from the Gotland study. *Lancet, 345,* 524.

Yesavage, J. A., Brink, T. L., Rose, T. L., & Adey, M. (1983). The geriatric depression rating scale: comparison with other self-report and psychiatric rating scales. In T. Crook, S. Ferris, & R. Bartus (Editors), *Assessment in geriatric psychopharmacology* (pp. 153–165). New Canaan, CT: Mark Powley Associates.

PART II

Treatment of Alcohol/Drug Misuse

6

Identification and Treatment of Alcohol Use Disorders in Older Adults

Michael Fleming

The goal of this chapter is to provide clinicians with clinical protocols that will help them take care of older adults. The protocols are based on the best evidence available. Unless otherwise stated the recommendations are based on studies conducted with adults over the age of 65. Since there is a paucity of prevention or treatment trials in persons over the age of 65, the author will try to clarify what we know and what we don't know about the prevention and treatment of alcohol use disorders in this population. Case examples are used to illustrate major points. The chapter is divided into seven sections: epidemiology and health effects, types of older drinkers, the new public health paradigm, identification, brief intervention, motivational interviewing, and pharmacotherapy.

Epidemiology and Health Effects

Prevalence studies suggest that 10%–12% of men and 2–5% of women over the age of 65 drink above the recommended limits of alcohol use (>1–2 drinks/day or >3–4 drinks per drinking occasion). Figures 6.1 and 6.2 present data from a large study conducted in 22 primary care practices in 10 counties in southern Wisconsin (Fleming et al., 1997). The

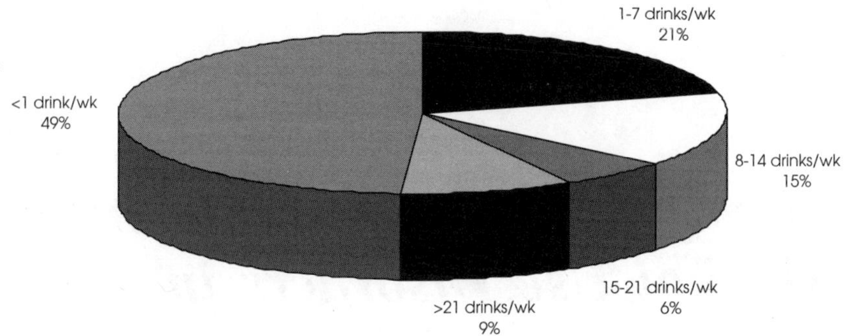

Figure 6.1 12-Month prevalence in primary care: Men ages 65-75

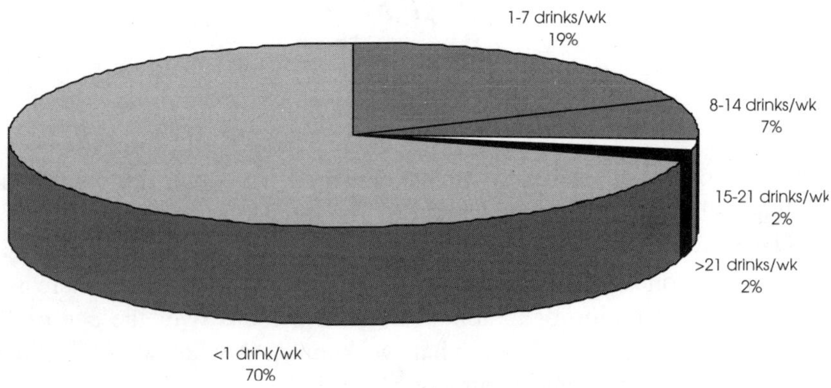

Figure 6.2 12-Month prevalence in primary care: Women ages 65-75

pie charts show varying levels of alcohol use in persons 66–75. As one can see, there is a marked gender difference in levels of use between men and women. Nearly 15% of male drinkers use alcohol above recommended limits. Based on these data the average primary care physician with 500 older adult men and women in his/her practice can expect that 40 to 50 of those patients will drink above recommended limits, about one patient in ten.

Alcohol use disorders are common in clinical settings and implicated in many health problems in older adults. The adverse effects of alcohol are dose-related and can occur in the absence of alcoholism. (See chapter 2 for Oslin's discussion of these issues.) The majority of these effects occur in nondependent problem drinkers. These adverse effects include: (a) falls and injuries; (b) medication adherence issues; (c) mental health problems such as depression, anxiety, suicide, and family violence; (d) mental status changes such as confusion, cognitive loss, and delirium; (e) cardiovascular illness such as hypertension, heart disease, and peripheral vascular occlusion; (f) endocrine illnesses such as glucose intolerance; (g) breast, esophageal, and colon cancer; (h) neurological problems such as peripheral neuropathy, strokes, ataxia, and dementia; and (i) gastrointestinal illness such as diarrhea, incontinence, liver failure, and abdominal pain (Stinson, 1989).

Alcohol also affects treatment for other problems and interacts with many commonly used medications. Treatment of hypertension, diabetes, heart disease, and depression is difficult in older adults who use alcohol on a regular basis. Clinically significant alcohol-medication interactions occur with (a) sedative-hypnotic drugs (e.g., oversedation with benzodiazepines); (b) antidepressants (e.g., cardiac problems with tricyclics); (c) antibiotics (e.g., toxicity issues with erythromycin and isoniazide); (d) anesthetic agents (e.g., accelerated metabolism with pentobarbital); (e) H2-blockers (e.g., higher blood alcohol levels with cimetidine and cisapride); (f) anticoagulants (e.g., accelerated metabolism with anticoagulants like Coumadin® and antiseizure medications such as Dilantin®); and (g) narcotics (e.g., cognitive effects of alcohol and morphine).

Alcohol and drug withdrawal can severely compromise post-operative care. Delirium tremens following repair of hip fractures in older adults is one of the more common reasons for referral to hospital-based alcohol consult services. Alcohol use can also complicate care in acute care settings such as emergency departments, coronary care units, burn units, and trauma life-support centers. Patients in active withdrawal are at greater risk for increasing the severity of myocardial ischemia and respiratory failure with pneumonia.

Types of Older Drinkers

The following case examples encountered in the author's practice illustrate the different types of drinkers. These include low-risk drinkers, at-risk drinkers, problem drinkers, and dependent drinkers.

Low-Risk Older Adult Drinkers

Low-risk older adult drinkers drink fewer than 1–2 drinks/day, do not drink more than 3–4 drinks per drinking occasion, and do not drink in high risk situations (e.g., driving a motor vehicle, before surgery, or while on medication that interacts with alcohol).

> Michael is a 70-year-old retired physician who drinks 3–4 times per week with friends. He rarely drinks more than 3 drinks/occasion. He doesn't like to become intoxicated, and never drives his car until the alcohol is out of his system. He has some mild hypertension but has no risk factors (e.g., no family history or history of alcohol or drug problems in the past) for developing alcohol-related problems.

At-Risk Older Adult Drinkers

At-risk older adult drinkers are defined as men and women who drink more than 1–2 drinks per day and/or more than 3–4 drinks per occasion. They are at risk for alcohol-related problems such as trauma, accidents, depression, and other effects, but like persons with a mild elevation in blood pressure or cholesterol, they may never experience adverse health effects related to these conditions. The following are examples of patients at risk for alcohol-related problems but who have so far avoided any serious problems.

> Iga is a 65-year-old school teacher who drinks two to three glasses of wine with dinner daily with her husband. Her use pattern has not changed since she retired 10 years ago. She has had no problems with her level of use, never gets drunk, and has no history of loss of control. She has no family history of alcohol problems and drinks because she enjoys the taste.

> Walter is a 70-year-old retired construction worker who drinks 2 or 3 beers nearly every day. He has no history of alcohol-related events and has not changed his use pattern in 20 years. He drank more heavily in his 20s but rarely drinks more than three beers at one sitting. He has not been drunk in 5 years. He is beginning to have some health problems and his physician has asked him to cut down on his alcohol use.

Older Adult Problem Drinkers

Older adult problem drinkers are defined as men and women who have developed one or more alcohol-related problems such as a "Driving

Under the Influence of Alcohol" (DUI) charge, medical complications, family problems, or other behavioral consequences. A problematic user may have experienced a single alcohol-or drug-related event, or may have developed more severe problems. Other terms used to describe this type of drinker are alcohol abuse and harmful drinkers.

John is a 66-year-old retired truck driver who drinks 4–5 beers 2 or 3 times per week. He was recently treated in the emergency room for a head injury secondary to a fall after he reportedly slipped on a patch of ice outside his home. He gets drunk about once a month and occasionally drives himself home while intoxicated. He uses alcohol to be sociable and has always been able to stop. The emergency department physician has told him to limit his alcohol use to 1–2 drinks per occasion and to see his regular provider if he has any problems cutting down.

Manuel is a 70-year-old farmer who drinks 3–4 beers nearly every day when he has finished his farm chores. His blood pressure was elevated and he developed chronic epigastric pain that responded to ranitidine. While he does not get visibly drunk, his children and grandchildren have been complaining about his heavy alcohol use and have asked him to stop. Blood pressure measurements over a 3-month period were elevated ranging from 160/110 to 140/98. A laboratory exam revealed an elevated GGT (gamma-glutamyl transferase), a liver function test. He remains abstinent 6 months after his physician and family confronted him. His blood pressure problem and epigastric pain have resolved.

Older Adult Alcohol-Dependent

Older adult alcohol-dependent (alcoholic) patients are those who have evidence of loss of control, preoccupation with use, family conflict, employment issues, blackouts, legal problems or other adverse effects, continued use despite health problems, and in some cases physical dependence (e.g., tolerance or withdrawal). In order to make a DSM-IV diagnosis of alcohol dependence patients are expected to meet at least three of seven DSM-IV criteria within the last 12–month period. A case example in primary care follows:

Irena is a 62-year-old widowed professional. In the past 2 years she has had two serious motor vehicle accidents while she was drinking. She drinks daily after work and sometimes at lunch. She occasionally drinks in the morning to get over a hangover and has experienced blackouts at least once per month. She drinks up to 10 drinks a day. Her friends have offered to drive her home but she refuses their help. She is a hard-working district attorney who was nominated to serve as an appellate court judge. She drinks alone and at parties. She has no other medical, mental health, family, or social problems. The ED physician confronted her at the time of one accident, but she denied any problem. The next year, while intoxicated, she was involved in an accident involving a fatality.

The New Public Health Paradigm?

The alcohol treatment field is moving toward a "harm reduction public health paradigm" and away from an exclusive focus on abstinence-based programs as the only legitimate goal of treatment. The harm reduction paradigm focuses on reducing alcohol use to low-risk levels, based on the observation that most problems related to alcohol use occur in persons who are not alcohol dependent. Most people who experience alcohol-related accidents, health problems, or family difficulties do not meet criteria for alcoholism; rather, they simply drink too much, often in high-risk situations (Graham, 1998; Institute of Medicine, 1990).

Most people with alcohol problems are not alcohol dependent but rather drink above recommended limits (at-risk drinker) or are experiencing some problems related to their alcohol use. Figure 6.3 sum-

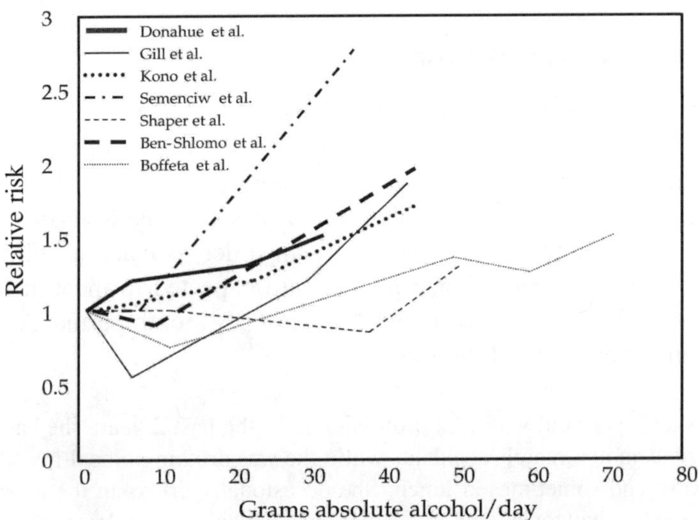

Figure 6.3 Strokes: Data from 7 Studies of Men (includes incidence & death)
Note. P. Anderson, et al. Personal communication, 1993. Reprinted with permission.

marizes the findings of a number of studies to illustrate the relationship of alcohol use to risk of stroke. As one can see, persons who drink more than 4 drinks per day (about 40 grams absolute alcohol) have a twofold risk of developing stroke. If we can reduce the level of use to 1–2 drinks the risk returns to baseline (Anderson, 1993).

The public health paradigm has important implications for the U.S. health care system. In the past, the physician's role was to identify persons with alcoholism and refer them for specialized treatment. Research conducted over the past 10 years has demonstrated that the role of providers has changed. A number of alcohol screening tests are available that are sensitive and specific for older adults (Adams, 1996). Clinical trials have shown the effectiveness of brief physician advice in reducing alcohol use and associated problems in problem drinkers (Fleming, 1997, 1999). The ability of primary care providers to follow patients and family members over a long period of time places them in a unique position to intervene and support the behavioral changes necessary to reduce the consequences of problem drinking. New medications such as opioid blocking agents (naltrexone), glutamate receptor antagonists (Acamprosate), and serotonin reuptake inhibitors (sertraline) are also expected to significantly add to the treatment options available (Garbutt, 1999).

Identification of Alcohol Use Disorders: Screening and Assessment

Figure 6.4 summarizes one approach to identifying and treating patients who have an alcohol use disorder. As one can see, the approach involves four steps. The first is to ask and screen. The second is to assess persons who screen positive. The third step is to conduct a brief intervention to have the patient cut down, prescribe medication, or refer the patient for treatment. The fourth is the follow-up and continuing care. The rest of this chapter focuses on these recommendations.

A number of alcohol screening instruments have been tested and validated in clinical settings for older adults. While researchers have proposed a number of theoretical reasons why older adults may require different questions than young adults, research has not borne this out. There are no specific questions found to work better in older adults. Screening questions that work well in general primary care samples of older adults include questions on quantity and frequency of alcohol consumption, binge drinking, and the four CAGE questions.

C = Have you ever felt you ought to Cut down on your drinking?
A = Have people Annoyed you by criticizing your drinking?
G = Have you felt bad or Guilty about your drinking?
E = Have you ever had an Eye-opener drink first thing in the morning to steady your nerves or get rid of a hangover?

These questions can be administered by direct interview as part of routine clinical care, by self-administered questionnaire, or by computer. Screening questionnaires developed specifically for pencil and paper or computer administration include the Alcohol Use Disorder Identification Test (AUDIT), the Health Screening Survey (HSS), PRIME-MD, and the geriatric version of the MAST.

Quantity and frequency questions, as recommended in the National Institute on Alcohol Abuse and Alcoholism's *Physicians' Guide to Helping Patients With Alcohol Problems* (NIAAA, 1995), are the current standard of practice used by the majority of physicians. These questions include:

1. Do you drink alcohol including beer, wine, or distilled spirits?
2. On average, how many days per week do you drink alcohol?
3. On a typical day when you drink, how many drinks do you have?
4. What is the maximum number of drinks you had on any given day in the past month?

1 Standard US drink = 11 grams absolute alcohol such as:
- 1 12oz. domestic beer (4% alcohol)
- 1 4–5oz. glass table wine (10–12% alcohol)
- 1 cocktail containing 1–1.5oz. alcohol

These questions have a number of strengths and comprise the only alcohol screening test that provides an estimate of alcohol-related risk. For example, older men who drink 4 or more standard US drinks/day have a twofold risk of developing stroke and liver failure compared with men who drink 1–2 standard drinks per day. (See Figure 6.3.) Quantity/frequency questions are sensitive, have a low rate of false-positive responses, are easy to score, and can be incorporated into a routine physician practice with minimal cost and effort (Adams, 1996). Underreporting, especially in persons who are alcohol dependent, cognitively impaired, or intoxicated can be minimized with appropriate interview techniques (a direct and nonjudgmental approach), collaborative reports (family member reports and medical record review), and laboratory tests (Breathalyzer, blood alcohol levels, gamma-glutamyl transferase [GGT], carbohydrate deficient transferrin [CDT]). Once a patient screens positive, clinicians may want to do a more thorough assessment to develop a treatment plan. Detailed information on screening is included in Oslin's chapter 2 on assessment.

Brief Intervention

Brief interventions are time-limited, patient-centered counseling strategies that focus on changing behavior and increasing medication compliance. Brief intervention is not unique to the treatment of alcohol problems; in fact, these counseling strategies are widely used by physicians and other health care professionals for other changing behaviors. For example, this method is routinely used to help patients change dietary habits, or for weight reduction, smoking cessation, cholesterol or blood pressure reduction, and improved adherence to prescription medications. While the focus of this chapter is on changing alcohol use, it is important to acknowledge that physicians use this technique daily for a variety of health care problems. The following information is a very brief review of the evidence. A recent report in the NIAAA journal *Alcohol Research & Health* provides a more comprehensive review of the subject (Fleming & Manwell, 1999).

The clinical elements of brief intervention for the prevention and treatment of alcohol problems vary across trials and clinical programs. However, a number of common elements can be identified:

Assessment: "Tell me about your drinking?" "What does your family or partner think about your drinking?" "Have you had any problems related to your alcohol use?" "What do you think about your drinking?" "Have you ever been concerned about how much you drink?"

Direct feedback: "As your doctor/therapist I am concerned about how much you drink and how it is affecting your health." "The car accident is a direct result of your alcohol use."

Contracting, negotiating, and goal setting: "You need to reduce your drinking. What do you think about cutting down to three drinks 2–3 times per week?" "I would like you to use these diary cards to keep track of your drinking over the next 2 weeks. We will review these at your next visit."

Behavioral modification techniques: "Here is a list of situations when people drink and sometimes lose control of their drinking. Let's talk about ways you can avoid these situations."

Self-help directed bibliotherapy: "I would like you to review this booklet and bring it with you at your next visit. It would be very helpful if you would complete some of the exercises in this guide."

Follow-up and reinforcement (establishing a plan for supportive phone calls and follow-up visits). "I would like you to schedule a follow-up appointment in 1 month to review your diary cards and I'll answer any questions you might have."

The number and duration of brief intervention sessions have varied by trial and setting. The classic brief intervention performed by a physician or nurse usually lasts for 5–10 minutes and is repeated 1–3 times over a 6- to 8-week period. Other trials that utilized therapists, social workers or psychologists as the interventionist usually had 30- to 60-minute counseling sessions for 1–6 visits. Some trials developed manuals or scripted workbooks. Others studies left it up to the interventionist to decide how to conduct the intervention based on a training program. Only one study was specifically conducted on a sample of older adults (Fleming, 1999).

Over the last 30 years there have been dozens of trials that have examined the efficacy of brief intervention (Bien, 1993; Wilk, 1997). The majority of these trials were conducted in samples of male patients, ages 18–70. There is limited evidence on the efficacy of brief intervention in older adults. While the majority of the trials included older adults, none, with the exception of Project GOAL, had large enough samples to conduct a meaningful analysis of this group. There is a second trial focused on older adults that is in the analysis phase at the University of Michigan (Barry, 2000). The following is a brief summary of the literature on the effectiveness of brief intervention literature:

Brief intervention counseling delivered by primary care providers, therapists, and research staff can decrease alcohol use for at least 1 year in nondependent drinkers in primary care clinics, managed care settings, hospitals, and research settings. (Bien, 1993; Fleming et al., 1997, 1999; Gentilello, 1999; Kahan, 1995; Marlatt, 1998; Ockene, 1999; WHO, 1996; Wilk, 1997). In positive trials, reductions in alcohol use varied from 10% to 30% between the brief intervention (brief talk therapy) and usual care control groups.

The effect size for men and women is similar (Fleming, 1997; Ockene, 1999; Wallace, 1988; WHO, 1996).

The effect size for persons over the age of 18 is similar for all age groups including older adults (Fleming et al., 1997, 1999; Marlatt, 1998; Monti, 1999; Ockene, 1999; Wallace, 1988; WHO, 1996).

Brief intervention can reduce subsequent health care utilization (Fleming, 1997; Gentilello, 1999; Israel, 1996; Kristenson, 1983). Project TrEAT (Trial for Early Alcohol Treatment) (Fleming, 1997) and Kristenson found reductions in emergency room visits and hospital days. Gentilello found reductions in hospital readmissions. Israel reported reductions in physician office visits.

Brief intervention can reduce alcohol-related harm. A number of studies found a reduction in laboratory tests such as GGT levels (Israel, 1996; Kristenson, 1983; Nillsen, 1991; Wallace, 1988), sick days (Chick, 1985; Kristenson, 1983), and drinking and driving (Fleming, unpublished; Monti, 1999).

Brief intervention may reduce mortality (Fleming, unpublished; Kristenson, 1983). These trials found twice as many deaths in the control group as in the experimental group.

Brief intervention may reduce health care and societal costs. An analysis of 12–month outcome data for Project TrEAT found a benefit-cost ratio of 5.6 to 1 for health care and societal costs (Fleming, 2000). Cost estimates performed by Holder (1995) using indirect data reported a cost saving of 1.5 to 1.

The authors will also review two trials conducted by the author (Fleming et al., 1997, 1999): Projects TrEAT and GOAL. Project TrEAT (Trial for Early Alcohol Treatment) is the largest brief intervention trial conducted in the U.S. health care system in community-based primary care practices. The trial was designed to replicate the Medical Research Council trial conducted in Great Britain. Physicians were recruited through the Wisconsin Research Network, local community hospitals, managed care organizations, and personal contacts. Sixty-four physicians from 17 clinics participated: 46 male and 18 female physicians, with a mean age of 46 and a mean of 13 years in practice. Seven hundred seventy-four men and women ages 18 to 65 years were randomized to a control group or a provider-delivered brief intervention group.

Major inclusion criteria included men who drank between 14 and 50 drinks per week, women who drank between 12 and 50 drinks per week, no evidence of alcohol dependence, and no alcohol treatment in the past 12 months. Seven hundred twenty-three subjects completed the 12–month follow-up interview, for a 93.4% follow-up rate. The major alcohol use outcome variables were average drinks per week, binge drinking, and excessive drinking. Large decreases were found for all alcohol use variables in all groups at 6 and 12 months. The greatest reductions occurred in the female experimental group, where use decreased 47% at 12 months (14.8 drinks per week down to 8.08 drinks/week). The difference between the female intervention group and the control group was significant for seven-day alcohol use (t=3.7; p<.001). Preliminary analysis suggests a possible treatment effect for days of hospitalization but not for emergency room visits. There was a difference in the use of hospital days at 6 and 12 months after the intervention for both men (chi-square=29.55, p<.01) and women (chi-square=10.98; p<.05).

Project GOAL (Guiding Older Adult Lifestyles) was designed to test the efficacy of brief physician advice in problem drinkers over the age of 65. It is the first brief intervention trial focused on older adults. It followed the same research protocols as Project TrEAT. Forty-three physicians from 24 community-based primary care practices located in eight Wisconsin counties were recruited and trained. Of the 6,073 patients screened for problem drinking, 105 males and 53 females met inclusion criteria (n=158) and were randomized into a control (n=71) or intervention group (n=87). One hundred forty-six subjects (92.4%) participated in the 12–month follow-up procedures. The 12–month follow-up indicated a significant reduction in seven-day alcohol use (t=3.77; p<.001), episodes of binge drinking (t=2.68, p<.005), and frequency of excessive drinking (t=2.65; p<.005). This is one of the few brief intervention trials where there were no pre-post randomization changes in drinking in the control group. No significant changes in health status were demonstrated; there were too few utilization events at 12 months to estimate differences between groups (Fleming, 1999).

Motivational Counseling

Table 6.1 presents the "stages of change" model. This model was developed by Prochaska and DiClemente (1992) to help clinicians deal with patients who are resistant and ambivalent about change. Strategies to help

Table 6.1 Stages of Change Model

Stage	Description	Counseling Objectives
Precontemplation	Not considering change	Identify patient's goals Provide information Bolster self-efficacy
Contemplation	Ambivalent about change	Develop discrepancy between goals and behavior Elicit self-motivational statements
Determination	Cognitively committed to change (made a decision to change now or soon)	Strengthen commitment to change Plan strategies for change
Action	Involved in change (began changing behaviors)	Identify and manage new barriers Recognize relapse or impending relapse
Maintenance	Behavior change is stable, but relapse is possible	Assure stability of change Foster personal development
Relapse	Undesired behaviors recur	Identify relapse Reestablish self-efficacy and commitment to change Learn from experience, develop new behavioral strategies
Termination	Change is very stable	Assure stability of change

patients in the different stages are presented. While this model has not been widely tested on older adults who have problems with alcohol use, the author has found these concepts and strategies to be very helpful in motivating patients to change (Fleming & Brown, 1999).

Stage 1: Precontemplation

Working with patients who are not ready to change

Barrier: Lack of Information—"I Never Thought About It. Why Should I?"

1. Assess the patient's understanding
   a. Explore the patient's explanatory model, i.e., for not considering change in drinking
   b. Identify the source and reasons for the patient's explanatory model

   c. Convey respect for the patient's explanatory model
2. Establish the patient's receptivity to additional information
   a. Check for interest in additional information
   b. Minimize distractions such as noise, time constraints, and other agenda items
3. Deliver the information
   a. Explain the information in small, digestible chunks
   b. Avoid jargon; use language appropriate to the patient's education, culture, and your comfort
   c. Periodically check for understanding by the patient; for complicated information, ask the patient to restate the information
4. Assess the patient's reaction
   a. Assess the patient's level of belief
   b. Assess the patient's view of the relevance and the implications of the new information

Barrier: Low Self-Efficacy—"I'd Like to Change, But I Can't."

1. Explore the origins of the low self-efficacy
   a. Previous failed attempts to change, or relapses
   b. Low self-esteem/self-worth—depression, other stigmatized conditions (e.g., substance abuse, eating disorders, obesity), previous or current abuse or violence, dysfunction in the patient's family of origin, personality disorders
2. Assess for reasons for relapses and reframe failures as learning experiences
   a. Normalize repeated relapses
3. Assess for other personal strengths and assert likelihood that patient can succeed
   a. Reframe the previous experiences; build a sense of self-efficacy
4. Provide or refer for treatment of an underlying psychiatric disorder or family dysfunction

Barrier: Contentment With the Present—"Things Are Fine Just the Way They Are."

1. Delineate the patient's views on the beneficial aspects of the behavior, i.e., continuing present drinking level
2. Ask the patient about the less beneficial aspects of the behavior.

3. Explore the patient's general goals—short-term and long-term.
4. Invite consideration regarding the compatibility between the patient's behavior and goals.

Stage 2: Contemplation

Working with patients who are thinking about taking some action

1. Express empathy
   a. Demonstrate acceptance without judging, criticizing, or blaming
   b. Practice skillful reflective listening
   c. Recognize ambivalence as normal
2. Develop discrepancy
   a. Help the patient develop an awareness of the important consequences and risks of the behavior
   b. Help the patient realize and amplify discrepancies between present behavior and broader goals as they impact motivation for change
   c. Have the patient present the arguments for change
3. Avoid argumentation
   a. Avoid prompting the patient to argue against change; don't argue for change
   b. Avoid labeling
   c. Interpret resistance by the patient as a signal to change strategies
4. Roll with resistance
   a. Reframe patients' statements slightly to create new momentum toward change
   b. Acknowledge reluctance and ambivalence as natural and understandable
   c. Engage the patient in problem solving—it's not your job to find the solutions
   d. Remember—it's ultimately the patient's decision
5. Support self-efficacy
   a. Support the patient's belief in his/her ability to succeed with the task
   b. Maintain that the patient is responsible for choosing and carrying out change
   c. Foster hope by presenting a range of alternative approaches

Stage 3: Determination

Working with patients already determined to change

1. Reinforce and strengthen commitment to change
   a. Reinforce the potential benefits of change
   b. Bolster self-efficacy
2. Help the patient develop a plan to change
   a. Identify what has and has not worked previously
   b. Identify the internal and external triggers for the behavior—consider moods; stresses; special occasions and celebrations; times of the day, week, month, or year; exposures to persons, places, or things
   c. Seek the patient's ideas about strategies for avoiding or dealing with the triggers
   d. If necessary, provide menus of strategic options from which the patient may choose
   e. Through questions, and perhaps gentle advice, help the patient foresee possible weaknesses in the plan
   f. When appropriate, suggest a focus on social supports, self-reward, and environmental change
   g. Honor the patient's decisions about the plan
   h. Review the plan, ensuring that it is concrete and specific
   i. Set an implementation date
   j. Set a contingency plan for possible difficulties
3. Make statements of partnership; reinforce benefits of change; bolster self-efficacy
4. Arrange follow-up

Stage 4: Action

Working with patients already taking steps toward change

A. Review the effectiveness of the previous strategies for change
1. Positives
   a. Identify the strategies that are working well and reinforce the patient's efforts
   b. Identify and reinforce any realized benefits of change

   c. Identify any disadvantages of change—what is missing and how can it be replaced without resuming the target behavior, i.e., increasing drinking
2. Potential to improve the previous strategies
   a. Identify the strategies that are not working well
   b. Identify the times that have been most difficult
   c. Identify "slips" (short-lived, limited resumptions of the increased drinking) and relapse
3. Identify any new or future potential challenges to behavior change—consider moods; stresses; special occasions and celebrations; times of the day, week, month, or year; exposures to persons, places, or things; overconfidence
4. Develop a plan for dealing with the current and anticipated challenges
   a. Seek the patient's ideas about strategies for avoiding or dealing with the triggers
   b. If necessary, provide menus of strategic options from which the patient may choose
   c. Through questions, and perhaps gentle advice, help the patient foresee possible weaknesses in the plan
   d. When appropriate, suggest a focus on social supports, self-reward, and environmental change
   e. Honor the patient's decisions about the plan
   f. Review the plan, ensuring that it is concrete and specific
   g. Set an implementation date
   h. Set a contingency plan for possible difficulties
5. Make statements of partnership; reinforce benefits of change; bolster self-efficacy
6. Arrange follow-up

Stage 5: Maintenance

Working with patients who have recently achieved drinking goals

1. Ensure that the behavioral change is stable
2. Identify goals for overall personal satisfaction—consider health, family and other interpersonal relationships, community, career, religion, and spirituality

3. Develop a plan for progressing toward personal development goals
   a. Seek the patient's ideas about strategies for avoiding or dealing with the triggers
   b. If necessary, provide menus of strategic options from which the patient may choose
   c. Through questions, and perhaps gentle advice, help the patient foresee possible weaknesses in the plan
   d. Honor the patient's decisions about the plan
   e. Review the plan, ensuring that it is concrete and specific
   f. Set an implementation date
   g. Set a contingency plan for possible difficulties

Stage 6: Relapse

Working with patients in relapse

1. Reinforce the normalcy of relapse
2. Bolster self-efficacy and self-esteem
3. Identify the precipitant(s) for the relapse
4. Attempt to reframe relapse as a potential learning experience
5. "Restage" the patient (has he/she returned to the stage of Precontemplation, Contemplation, Determination, or Action?)

Pharmacotherapy

Patients who do not respond to brief intervention or self-help groups such as AA, and alcohol-dependent patients benefit from pharmacological management. Studies specifically conducted with older adults are noted. Effective medications for the treatment of alcohol problems include disulfiram (Antabuse®), naltrexone (ReVia®), calcium acetylhomotaurinate (Acamprosate®), serotonin reuptake inhibitors, and tricyclic antidepressants (Litten & Allen, 1991; Mason, 1996; Meyer, 1989; Sellers, 1981).

Disulfiram is the most commonly used medication to deter patients from drinking alcohol during recovery. While the efficacy of this medication is variable, disulfiram is widely used throughout the world in tablet and implant form. If patients who are alcohol dependent take disulfiram on a daily basis, it can be an effective deterrent. Spousal monitoring can significantly increase adherence and reduce rates of relapse. Disulfiram inhibits several enzyme systems including aldehyde dehydrogenase (ADH) and dopamine-beta-hydroxylase. This medication has to be used with caution in older adults with a history of heart disease since it may cause liver disease and may aggravate depression.

Naltrexone is an opioid receptor antagonist that binds primarily to mu-type opioid receptors. It was initially found to reduce alcohol use in laboratory animals, and subsequent randomized controlled trials have found reductions in alcohol use and craving in alcohol-dependent persons. The drug does not appear to be effective when used without counseling and other standard treatment. It is viewed as a treatment adjunct rather than as a replacement for traditional treatment. The effectiveness of naltrexone in nondependent problem drinkers is not known. There is one study reported in older adults suggesting naltrexone is safe and can reduce craving in this population (Oslin, 1997).

The most common side effect is nausea (10%), which usually resolves in a few days. Vomiting is uncommon. Idiosyncratic reactions include fatigue, dizziness, restlessness, and insomnia. In an open label trial with 530 subjects, 5% developed symptoms similar to narcotic withdrawal including abdominal cramps, joint pain, myalgia, and nasal stuffiness. It is important to inform patients taking narcotics that they should not take narcotics when taking naltrexone, as they will go into acute withdrawal.

Calcium acetylhomotaurinate (Acamprosate®) is an orally available, nonmetabolized, modified amino acid that is not protein bound. It has a relative specificity for brain NMDA and GABA receptors, which themselves are involved in learning and anxiety relief. Alcohol has activity at NMDA receptors. Acamprosate® appears to act at glutamate receptors as a competitive antagonist and to decrease craving in alcohol-dependent persons. Eleven controlled placebo trials have been conducted in Europe; 10 demonstrated superior efficacy of Acamprosate® over placebo when the medication was combined with psychosocial treatment. Few patients over age 65 have been included in these trials. These trials used doses of up to 2000 mg per day for periods of up to 1 year with only one major side effect—diarrhea—in 10% of the cases. Unfortunately, small sample size, 40% to 60% loss to follow-up rates, and noncompliance with treatment compromised the scientific strength of these trials. The medication is expected to become available in the U.S. soon, where a number of trials are ongoing.

Animal studies have found lower concentrations of serotonin and its metabolites (5–HIAA) in cerebrospinal fluid in alcohol-dependent persons. As a result, researchers have proposed a number of methods to increase the amount and activity of serotonin in the brain. L-tryptophan, which is the amino acid precursor to serotonin, appears to have some effect in laboratory animals and may directly increase concentrations of serotonin. The serotonin receptor agonist, buspirone, has reduced alcohol use in small studies. The use of serotonin reuptake inhibitors to reduce craving is being intensively studied by pharmaceutical companies.

Serotonin reuptake inhibitors (e.g., fluoxetine, marketed as Prozac®) appear to enhance serotonin activity in the central nervous system. These drugs have been traditionally used to treat depression, panic attacks, low self-esteem, and obsessive compulsive disorders. A number of small clinical trials with zimelidine, citalopram, viqualine, and fluoxetine suggest a modest treatment effect in reducing alcohol use both in depressed heavy drinkers and depressed alcoholics. The effect size ranges from 10% to 26%; however, a number of serious design problems make it difficult to interpret the results. Their efficacy in nondepressed patients remains controversial. Common serotonin reuptake inhibitors such as Prozac® or Zoloft® are not currently recommended for alcohol abuse until larger trials have been conducted.

Summary

This chapter provides a summary of screening, assessment, and treatment methods for the care of older adults drinking above recommended levels of alcohol use. As described in Figure 6.4, all older adults should be screened for alcohol use at least every 2–3 years. Persons drinking above recommended limits should be assessed for alcohol problems and dependence. Brief intervention can be used to help patients reduce their drinking or become abstinent. Motivational interviewing can be helpful for patients who are resistant to or ambivalent about change. Pharmacotherapy provides physicians with new treatment options to help patients who have craving or mental health disorders. Clinicians have a wonderful

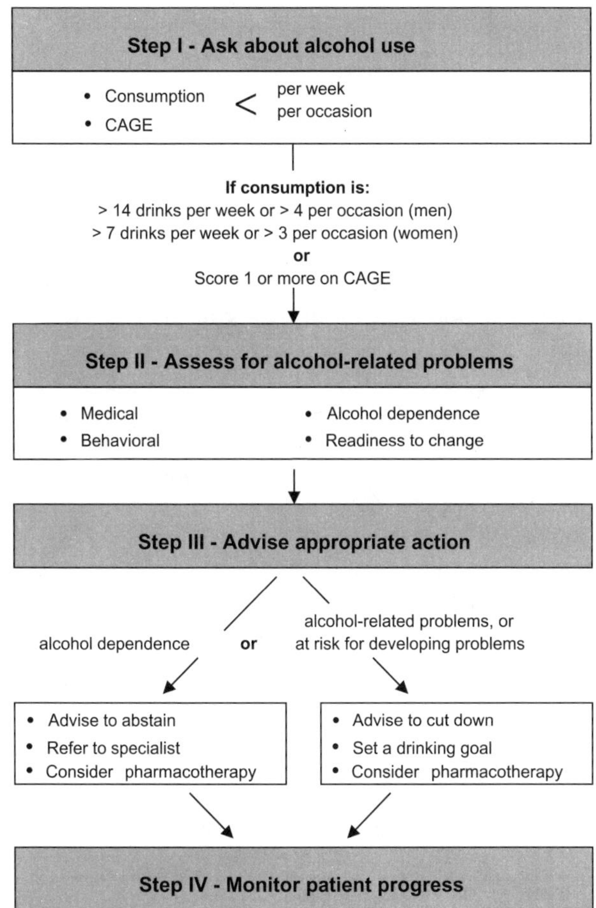

Figure 6.4 Steps for alcohol screening and brief intervention.

opportunity to prevent and treat alcohol problems in older adults using these methods.

References

Adams, W. L., Barry, K. L., & Fleming, M. F. (1996). Screening for problem drinking in older primary care patients. *Journal of the American Medical Association, 276*(24), 1964–1967.

Anderson P., Cremona A., Paton A., & Turner, C. (1993). The risk of alcohol. *Addiction, 88,* 1493–1508.

Babor T., Korner P., Wilber C., & Good, S. (1987). Screening and early intervention strategies for harmful drinkers: Initial lessons from the AMETHYST Project. *Austrian Drug Alcohol Review, 6,* 325–339.

Barry, K. L. (2000). Personal communication.

Bien, T. H., Miller, W. R., & Tonigan, J. S. (1993). Brief interventions for alcohol problems: A review. *Addiction, 88,* 315–335.

Buchsbaum, D. G., Buchanan, R. G., Welsh J., Centro, R. M., & Schnoll, S. H. (1992). Screening for drinking disorders in the elderly using the CAGE questionnaire. *Journal of the American Geriatrics Society, 40,* 662–665.

Chick J., Lloyd G., & Crombie, E. (1985). Counseling problem drinkers in medical wards: A controlled study. *British Medical Journal, 290,* 965–967.

DeHart, S. S., & Hoffmann, N. G. (1995). Screening and diagnosis of "alcohol abuse and dependence" in older adults. *International Journal of Addiction, 30*(13–14), 1717–1747.

Fleming, M. F., Mundt, M. P., French, M. T., Manwell, L. B., Stauffacher, E. A., & Barry, K. L. (2000). Benefit-cost analysis of brief physician advice with problem drinkers in primary care settings. *Medical Care, 38*(1), 7–18.

Fleming, M. F., Mundt, M. P., French, M. T., Manwell, L. B., & Stauffacher, E. A. Project TrEAT, a trial for early alcohol treatment: 4–year follow-up. Unpublished.

Fleming, M. F., & Manwell, L. B. (1999). Brief intervention in primary care settings. *Alcohol Research and Health, 232*), 128–137.

Fleming, M. F., & Brown, R. L. (1999). Motivational interviewing. In M. F. Fleming, & M. Murray (Editors), A medical education model for the prevention and treatment of alcohol use disorders. National Institutes of Health, National Institute on Alcohol Abuse and Alcoholism.

Fleming, M. F., Manwell, L. B., Barry, K. L., Adams W., Mundt., M., & Stauffacher, E. A. (1999). Brief physician advice for older adult problem alcohol drinkers: A randomized controlled trial. *Journal of Family Practice, 48*(5), 378–384.

Fleming, M. F., Barry, K. L., Manwell, L. B., Johnson K., & London, R. (1997). Brief physician advice for problem alcohol drinkers. A randomized controlled trial in community-based primary care practices. *Journal of the American Medical Association, 277,* 1039–1045.

Fleming, M. F., & Barry, K. L. (1991). A three-sample test of a masked alcohol screening questionnaire. *Alcohol and Alcoholism, 26,* 81–91.

Garbutt, J. C., West, S. L., Carey, T. S., Lohr, K. N., & Crews, F. T. (1999). Pharmacological treatment of alcohol dependence: A review of the evidence. *Journal of the American Medical Association, 281*(14), 1318–1325.

Gentilello, L. M., Rivara, F. P., Donovan, D. M., Jurkovich, G. J., Daranciang,

E., Dunn, C. W., Villaveces, A., Copass, M., & Riess, R. R. (1999). Alcohol interventions in a trauma center as a means of reducing the risk of injury recurrence. *Annals of Surgery, 230*(4), 437–480.

Graham, K., & Schmidt, G. (1998). The effects of drinking on health of older adults. *The American Journal of Drug and Alcohol Abuse, 24*(3), 465–481.

Holder, H. D., Miller, T. R., & Carina, R. T. (1995). *Cost savings of substance abuse prevention in managed care.* Rockville, MD: Substance Abuse and Mental Health Services Administration, Center for Substance Abuse Prevention (CSAP).

Institute of Medicine, Division of Mental Health and Behavioral Medicine. (1990). *Broadening the base of treatment for alcohol problems.* Washington, DC: National Academic Press.

Israel, Y., Hollander, O., Sanchez-Craig, M., Booker, S., Miller, V., Gingrich, R., & Rankin, J. G. (1996). Screening for problem drinking and counseling by the primary care physician-nurse team. *Alcoholism, Clinical and Experimental Research, 20,* 1443–1450.

Jones, T. V., Lindsey, B. A., Yount, P., Soltys, R., & Farani-Enayat, B. (1993). Alcoholism screening questionnaires: Are they valid in elderly medical outpatients? *Journal of General Internal Medicine, 8,* 674–678.

Kahan, M., Wilson, L., & Becker, L. (1995). Effectiveness of physician-based interventions with problem drinkers: A review. *Canadian Medical Association Journal, 152,* 851–859.

Kristenson, H., Ohlin, H., Hulten-Nosslin, M. B., Trell, E., & Hood, B. (1983). Identification and intervention of heavy drinking in middle-aged men: Results and follow-up of 24–60 months of long-term study with randomized controls. *Alcoholism, Clinical and Experimental Research, 7*(2), 203–209.

Litten, R., & Allen, J. (1991). Pharmacotherapies for alcoholism: Promising agents and clinical issues. *Alcoholism, Clinical and Experimental Research, 15*(4), 620–633.

Marlatt, G. A., Baer, J. S., Kivlahan, D. R., Dimeff, L. A., Larimer, M. E., Quigley, L. A., Somers, J. M., & Williams, E. (1998). Screening and brief intervention for high-risk college student drinkers: Results from a 2–year follow-up assessment. *Journal of Consulting and Clinical Psychology, 66,* 604–615.

Mason, B. J., Kocsis, J. H., Ritvo, E. C., & Cutler, R. B. (1996). A double-blind, placebo-controlled trial of desipramine for primary alcohol dependence stratified on the presence or absence of major depression. *Journal of the American Medical Association, 275*(10), 761–767.

Meyer, R. (1989). Prospects for a rational pharmacotherapy of alcoholism. *Journal of Clinical Psychiatry, 50,* 403–412.

Monti, P. M., Colby, S. M., Barnett, N. P., Spirito, A., Rohsenow, D. J., Meyers, M., Wooland, R., & Lewander, W. (1999). Brief intervention for harm reduction with alcohol-positive older adolescents in a hospital emergency department. *Journal of Consulting and Clinical Psychology, 67,* 989–994.

National Institute on Alcohol Abuse and Alcoholism. (1995). *The physicians' guide to helping patients with alcohol problems.* U.S. Department of Health and Human Services, Public Health Service, National Institutes of Health.

Nilssen, O. (1991). The Tromso Study: Identification of and a controlled intervention on a population of early-stage risk drinkers. *Preventive Medicine, 20,* 518–528.

Ockene, J. K., Adams, A., Hurley, T. G., Wheeler, E. V., & Hebert, J. R. (1999). Brief physician- and nurse practitioner-delivered counseling for high-risk drinkers: Does it work? *Archives of Internal Medicine, 159*(18), 2198–2205.

Oslin, D., Liberto, J. G., O'Brien, J., Krois, S., & Norbeck, J. (1997). Naltrexone as an adjunctive treatment for older patients with alcohol dependence. *American Journal of Geriatric Psychiatry, 5*(4), 324–332.

Prochaska, J. O., & DiClemente, C. C. (1992). Stages of change in the modification of problem behaviors. In M. Hersen, R. M. Eisler, & P. M. Miller (Editors), *Progress in behavior modification* (pp. 184–214). Sycamore, IL: Sycamore Press.

Sellers, E., Naranjo, C., & Peachey, J. (1981). Drugs to decrease alcohol consumption. *New England Journal of Medicine, 305,* 1255–1262.

Stinson, F. S., Dufour, M. C., & Bertolucci, D. (1989). Alcohol-related morbidity in the aging population. *Alcohol Health and Research World, 13*(1), 80–87.

Wallace, P., Cutler, S., & Haines, A. (1988). Randomised controlled trial of general practitioner intervention in patients with excessive alcohol consumption. *British Medical Journal, 297*(10), 663–668.

Wilk, A. I., Jensen, N. M., & Havighurst, T. C. (1997). Meta-analysis of randomized control trials addressing brief interventions in heavy alcohol drinkers. *Journal of General Internal Medicine, 12*(5), 274–83.

World Health Organization Brief Intervention Group. (1996). A cross-national trial of brief interventions with heavy drinkers. *American Journal of Public Health, 86*(7), 948–955.

7

Age-Specific Cognitive-Behavioral and Self-Management Treatment Approaches

Lawrence Schonfeld and Larry W. Dupree

Introduction

Once an older adult has been identified as having a serious substance abuse problem, the next step in the continuum of care is to refer that person to the appropriate treatment program. For those cases in which brief intervention (see chapter 6 in this volume) is not sufficient, admission to an outpatient or inpatient treatment program must be considered. Unfortunately, there are relatively few age-specific treatment programs in the United States, and only a handful of programs in Canada (Dupree & Schonfeld, in press). This makes referral to the appropriate treatment difficult, with most referral sources attempting to place the older adult in programs which mix younger and older substance abusers. This is illustrated by the fact that, at least in the U.S., less than 6% of individuals admitted to alcohol treatment programs are age 55 or older (National Institute on Drug Abuse and National Institute on Alcohol Abuse and Alcoholism, 1990), proportionally far less than their numbers within the general population.

When age-specific treatment can be offered, recommended characteristics for programs which treat the older substance abusers can be applied. In a recent Treatment Improvement Protocol ("TIP"), the expert panel recommended that older adults would benefit from: age-specific group treatment, a "supportive" rather than confrontational atmosphere, staff trained to work with older people, and a program which provides clients with the skills to address common triggers for drinking, including depression and loneliness, cognitive-behavioral treatment (CBT), and self-management (SM) approaches (Center for Substance Abuse Treatment, 1998). In this chapter, we describe how CBT/SM has been used with older substance abusers and provide case examples of the assessment and treatment planning process.

CBT/SM approaches are based on the Relapse Prevention (RP) model offered by Marlatt and Gordon (1985) which, in turn, is based on research stemming from interviews with individuals who relapsed following treatment. In most cases, relapses were preceded by intrapersonal events such as negative affect (e.g., feelings of depression, loneliness, tension, frustration), or interpersonal events such as conflicts with other people or social pressure to use alcohol or drugs. Thus, in the RP model, individuals faced with these high risk situations are likely to avoid alcohol or drugs if they have appropriate coping skills to address the situations. If they lack these skills, it results in poor self-efficacy or confidence in their ability to cope, leading to increased probability of a slip or lapse. This in turn leads to experiencing an abstinence violation effect, which increases the possibility of a full relapse.

Treatment programs which offer RP strategies usually employ CBT/SM approaches to teach clients the skills necessary to avoid relapse, relying on techniques such as cognitive-restructuring, thought-stopping/covert assertion, problem solving, self-monitoring and self-reinforcement techniques. Similar models have been used in age-specific treatment programs in Canada designed to enhance self-efficacy and teach the appropriate skills (Graham, Brett, & Baron, 1997; Saunders, Graham, Flower, & White-Campbell, 1992; West & Graham, 1999).

The RP approach to planning and implementing treatment begins with identification of each individual's high risk situations for substance use, teaching the individual to be aware of those triggers for use, and teaching appropriate skills to prevent relapse should these situations occur again after treatment. That first step involves behavior analysis of drinking or substance use through a structured interview in order to identify the antecedents which typically precede substance use as well as the consequences of use, especially those positive consequences which may serve to reinforce the use of that substance. We begin this discussion by describing the utility of identifying the components of a substance abuse behavior chain and diagramming those components for the benefit of the client's education about his/her use of alcohol or drugs.

The Substance Abuse Behavior Chain

The substance abuse behavior chain is really a diagrammatic timeline representing the individual's typical antecedents to the first use of alcohol or drugs on a typical day of use and the consequences or events which follow that first use. The components of the behavior chain are identified using a structured interview with the client which is later diagrammed for instructional purposes to teach the client to be aware of the triggers and consequences of his or her drinking or drug use. Originally developed in 1979 as a drinking behavior chain for use with late onset alcohol abusers in the Gerontology Alcohol Project ("GAP") by Dupree, Broskowski, and Schonfeld (1984), the drinking behavior chain was later modified as the substance use behavior chain, for use with individuals who abused one or more substances such as alcohol, illicit drugs, or prescription medications (Dupree & Schonfeld, 1996). Figure 7.1 illustrates the components of the substance abuse behavior chain moving along the time line of events from left to right.

In order to identify the components of the chain, staff members are trained to use a structured interview designed to identify the interactions with other people, the location, activities, cognitions, etc., which typically precede substance use, and the positive and negative consequences of that use. In the next section we describe two similar, structured interviews that have been used for identifying the components of the substance abuse behavior chain.

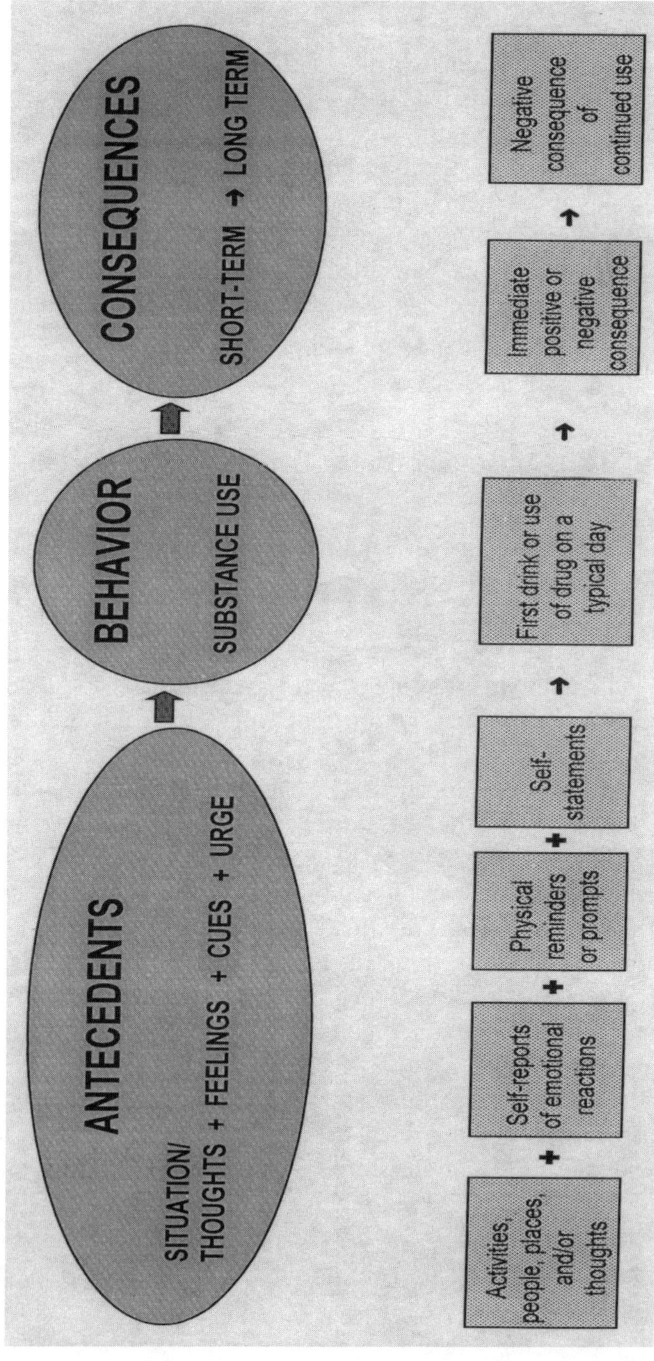

Figure 7.1 The substance abuse behavior chain.

Analysis of Drinking Behavior

In GAP, each newly admitted client was interviewed using the Gerontology Alcohol Project Drinking Profile (GAP-DP) to identify the antecedents, behavior, and consequences of substance use, i.e., the "A-B-Cs." The GAP-DP included questions concerning family history, treatment and substance use history, and recent drinking patterns (type of beverages, quantity, frequency, and typical pattern of use). The most critical questions for treatment planning purposes, however, were those which identified the most frequent antecedents to consuming the first drink on a typical day of drinking in the 30 days preceding the last drink prior to admission and the most frequent consequences of that first drink.

The questions on antecedents and consequences paralleled the timeline of the behavior chain shown in Figure 7.1. Categories of antecedents included situations and/or thoughts, feelings, cues, and urges (self-statements). Situations refer to the place or location where drinking would take place, activities in which he or she might have been engaged, and people with whom he/she drank. Most GAP clients reported being at home, alone, with no activities planned or engaging only in solitary activities such as watching television. This led to thinking about the past or about recent losses, which in turn frequently led to feelings of depression, sadness, loneliness, or boredom. As most people do not verbalize or even conceptualize, at least at admission to treatment, their emotions or feelings as precipitants for drinking, the structured interview serves as a useful tool to assist the staff member conducting the interview in identification of these covert behaviors, often enlightening the client as well. To this end, using the GAP-DP, the interviewer would ask each client to define what he or she meant by the response selected. For example, when describing feelings or emotional states prior to drinking, many clients in GAP selected "depressed" as the most frequent feeling just before taking a drink on a typical day. For each such response, the GAP staff member asked him or her "What were you depressed about?" and then recorded the client's response. This enabled staff to better identify the reasons for turning to alcohol. Many older GAP participants drank to alleviate depression. This is noteworthy since many of our GAP clients did not score high on depression inventories, but still frequently reported feeling depressed prior to the drink.

Proceeding along the time line within the behavior chain, if certain cues were present, they served as prompts or reminders to drink. Obvious cues may be seeing other people consuming alcohol, while less obvious cues may be certain times of the day or driving along certain routes which remind someone of the way to their neighborhood bar. Many of the GAP clients who reported feeling lonely and depressed, indicated that the time of day—especially late afternoon or early evening—was a common cue. Other cues included watching certain television programs, hearing certain kinds of music, receiving the Social Security check in the mail, seeing a neighborhood bar on the way home from shopping, etc.

The last component in the drinking behavior chain is the "urge." Rather than viewing the urge as a physiological response or related to cravings, in the GAP program the urge was seen as a self-statement such as "A cold beer would help me feel relaxed" or "I'll get even with my wife!" The urge is the last event occurring before the consumption of alcohol. Often, clients may not realize the nature of such self-statements until the questions in the structured interview, which deal with consequences of the first drink, are asked.

Regarding consequences after the first drink, the time line of the drinking behavior chain shown in Figure 7.1 identifies the short-term consequences following the first drink, referring to immediate consequences. Often these were positive consequences which served as reinforcers that maintain drinking. For example, alcohol was reinforcing because one expected to feel more relaxed, less depressed, more sociable, less lonely, etc.; and it occurred. In a few cases, short-term consequences were "negative" such as "I felt guilty about taking a drink" or "my wife yelled at me when she saw me starting to drink." With further progression of the time line, long-term consequences can be identified to explore how drinking negatively impacted one's life. Long-term consequences were always negative effects of continued and excessive drinking, including "I was worried about my health" or "I worry that my wife would leave me." Because long-term consequences lack the temporal contingency of drinking and adverse effect, they rarely prevent drinkers from avoiding alcohol. The questions regarding immediate, positive consequences can be reframed into the antecedent section on urges. Thus, consequences such as "I felt more relaxed after the first drink" or "I felt happier after the first drink" reveal antecedent urges to the drink such as tension or depression, respectively.

In GAP, once the interview was complete and the client's responses recorded, the staff member conducting the interview constructed the drinking behavior chain for that particular client using the responses provided. Each client was provided a typewritten copy of the antecedent and consequences for his/her review and use within the group treatment modules. In that way, clients would have prompts to use for group discussions and exercises.

Adaptation of the GAP-DP

As we admitted older adults into a successor program (the Substance Abuse Program for the Elderly), it soon became apparent that some older adults misused other substances such as prescription medications. For those cases, we developed a profile similar to the GAP-DP interview, but with questions altered to address the use of the medications. This profile will be illustrated later in this chapter in a case example.

Another adaptation of the GAP-DP was necessary when we were asked to consult with a California-based program for veterans. In 1996, we became involved in the development of an age-specific, CBT/SM program known as "GET SMART" (Geriatric Evaluation Team: Substance Misuse/Abuse Recognition and Treatment) at the VA Greater Los Angeles Healthcare System—West Los Angeles Healthcare Center. To accommodate a population of elderly veterans who were more likely to use multiple substances, we developed the Substance Abuse Profile for the Elderly and modified the treatment curriculum to address multiple substance use including illicit drugs, and sample situations pertinent to veterans (Dupree & Schonfeld, 1996). Despite differences in the demographics and types of substances used, there were many similarities between GET SMART patients and the GAP clients. Both groups tended to use substances at home, alone, and in response to negative affect—primarily feelings of depression, loneliness, sadness, etc.—and both groups tended to experience a positive affect immediately after use, usually feeling happy, relaxed, etc.

Treatment Planning

Following the identification of the substance abuse behavior chain, the next step in CBT/SM approaches is to plan and implement treatment so that each client's antecedent to drinking or drug use is addressed within the group treatment modules. In this section we describe how this process took place in GAP, the Substance Abuse Program for the Elderly, and more recently the GET SMART program.

The Gerontology Alcohol Project

GAP was the first age-specific program for older adults which utilized cognitive-behavioral and self-management approaches. The program offered at the Florida Mental Health Institute from 1979–1981 targeted late onset, older alcohol abusers from the Tampa Bay area of Florida. To be eligible for admission, clients had to be age 55 or older, with onset of the drinking problem occurring after age 50.

The GAP treatment involved a three-phase approach. In the first phase, each newly admitted client was assessed using the GAP-DP as described earlier. In the second stage, clients entered the first module called the "A-B-Cs" of drinking, designed to teach them to break down drinking behavior into Antecedents-Behavior-Consequences, with drinking being the targeted behavior ("B"). A module was a treatment group with a manual containing the session by session content, and methods for assessing level of knowledge or skills acquired (such as ratings of behavior rehearsals or quizzes). In the A-B-C module, information gathered from the GAP-DP was used to teach each person to identify his/her own antecedents and consequences, and learn which situations would become "high-risk situations" for alcohol consumption. Clients learned to identify their own antecedents and consequences using the information from the behavior chain.

Once GAP clients demonstrated through quizzes, rehearsal, and class exercises that they could master the knowledge of their "A-B-Cs," they entered the third phase of treatment, a series of "Alcohol Self-Management" modules addressing such antecedents as social pressure/drink refusal, anger/frustration, anxiety and tension, cues, urges, and slips. A variety of teaching techniques and CBT/SM approaches were used within these modules. Examples of these techniques included behavior rehearsal to sample situations read aloud by the group leader, lectures on the appropriate skills, covert rehearsals in which the client stated aloud what he or she would do if a covert behavior such as the urge occurred or if a slip occurred, learning how to record or self-monitor urges to drink and drinking behavior itself through weekly "drinking logs," relaxation techniques for coping with tension, general problem-solving skills, and cognitive restructuring and thought-stopping techniques for recognition of inaccurate negative self-statements and cognitions.

These and other related CBT/SM techniques were provided to staff within the written curriculum. That curriculum was written for paraprofessionals, since the typical staff member had a bachelors degree, rather than graduate level training or licensure in a counseling field. The text of the curriculum provided easy-to-follow, session-by-session lecture content, to ensure that treatment was being delivered uniformly, regardless of which staff member conducted the group, and irrespective of the staff member's background or level of education. The curriculum also provided quizzes, exercises with sample situations pertinent to older adults, and rating scales for staff to rate clients' behavior rehearsals. The quizzes and behavior rehearsal ratings also provided an objective measure of the mastery of the knowledge and skills taught. Thus, staff members serving as group leaders and case managers did not rely on guesswork to judge a client's success within modules, but instead, relied on objective measures of whether knowledge was gained and skills demonstrated.

The average length of stay in the active phase of the treatment program was 16 weeks. However, individual length of stay was determined by assessment within the treatment modules designed to attend to the individual's antecedents for abuse. Thus, a "successful completer" was one who acquired the behavioral skills necessary to preclude or terminate high risk/antecedent conditions, and could demonstrate such. Treatment modules were scheduled 5 days per week, but not all modules were offered each day. The various treatment modules were typically offered twice per week. Based upon the number of antecedent conditions needing attention, individuals could be assigned to multiple treatment modules that would in turn necessitate attendance more often than twice per week, should their assigned modules not occur on the same days.

Once a client successfully completed the modules as indicated by the assessments, he or she was eligible for successful discharge from the active phase of treatment, and was invited to enter the 12–month follow-up program. Follow-up consisted of visits and/or telephone contacts with the clients. Assessments used at discharge (drinking profile; scales to measure depression, self-esteem, anxiety, and social support) were administered during follow-up visits at 1, 3, 6, and 12 months post-discharge.

Over a 2-year period, GAP received 153 age and criteria appropriate referrals. Of those, 48 agreed to enter treatment, with 24 completing treatment and entering the follow-up phase. Results showed that three quarters of program completers maintained abstinence or goals of limited drinking over the 1-year follow-up, increased independent living skills, and increased the size of their social support network. In addition, there were significant improvements in ratings of clients' drinking behavior by significant others (e.g., family members).

Funding for GAP ended in 1981. However, in 1986, a subsequent treatment program, the Substance Abuse Program for the Elderly, was created (also at the Florida Mental Health Institute, University of South Florida) which employed the same treatment modules and strategies. That program admitted any older adult with a substance abuse problem, regardless of age of onset or type of substance used. Thus, we began to admit early onset alcohol abusers as well as people who misused prescription medications. Results from the latter program illustrated that older alcohol abusers, regardless of whether their drinking problems were considered early or late onset, had similar antecedents to alcohol use, and often to medication misuse, with negative affect and social isolation being the most common triggers for recent substance use (Schonfeld & Dupree, 1991).

The GET SMART Program

A modified version of the GAP curriculum was also implemented in an age-specific program for elderly veterans in Los Angeles. GET SMART started in 1991 as a program providing weekly support groups to veterans age 60 and older with substance abuse problems. In 1996, the program shifted to the use of CBT/SM approaches based on a modified curriculum from the GAP program. Patients served by GET SMART are voluntary admissions to substance abuse treatment, referred through medical units, outreach efforts, or self-referral. Participants are typically medically impaired and are frequently homeless or domiciliary based. About half are African American veterans.

The GET SMART curriculum is offered once a week for 16 weeks in group treatment format (Dupree & Schonfeld, 1996). All admissions are first interviewed using the Substance Abuse Profile for the Elderly, an adaptation of the GAP-DP which addresses the use or abuse of multiple substances such as alcohol, illicit drugs, and/or improper use of prescribed medications. The CBT/SM modules offered a similar program to GAP, teaching skills addressing social pressure, being at home alone, feelings of depression and loneliness, anxiety and tension, anger and frustration, cues for substance use, urges (self-statements), and slips or relapses. The GAP curriculum was modified to include sample situations used in group exercises and rehearsals pertinent to older veterans and to individuals using illicit drugs.

Recently, the results of the first 110 GET SMART admissions to the CBT/SM modules were described (Schonfeld et al., 2000). At admission, most participants were found to be veterans of the Korean War. Many were medically impaired, and more than a third were homeless. Half of the admissions were minorities (most being African Americans) for whom illicit drug use was higher than for Caucasians. Surprisingly, while alcohol was the most frequently used substance, 38% of the GET SMART patients used illicit drugs such as heroin or crack cocaine either in combination with alcohol (29%) or without alcohol (9%). Also about one-third of illicit drug users reported onset of a drug abuse problem after age 50.

Of the 110 admissions, 49 completed CBT/SM groups and 61 dropped out of treatment. Six-month telephone follow-up interviews revealed much higher rates of abstinence among those completing treatment than those not completing. Follow-up of program participants is continuing at this writing.

In summary, structured interviews such as those used in the GAP, Substance Abuse Program for the Elderly, and the GET SMART programs address clients' needs without relying on the use of labels, confrontation, or accusations. Instead, the interview process "matter-of-factly" gathers information about many problems (e.g., feelings precipitating drinking; consequences of drinking). Rather than force individuals into treatment decisions, the client is treated as a "co-therapist" by negotiating drinking goals and changes in behaviors with the staff member. Thus, with such an approach the information revealed by the client becomes useful information for treatment planning, reviewing progress in treatment, and reviewing what happened when a slip occurred.

Follow-Up and Aftercare

Some form of follow-up was offered in each of the CBT/SM programs described in this chapter. Follow-up and aftercare provide important contacts with individuals who have completed treatment, especially within the first few months following discharge when relapse is most likely to occur. Marlatt and Gordon (1985) demonstrated the likelihood of relapse during the first 90 days after treatment, mostly in response to intrapersonal events such as negative affect, and interpersonal events such as social pressure or conflicts with others. Our research indicates that prior to admission, negative affect is more likely to lead to drinking among the elderly than it is among younger substance abusers (Schonfeld, Dupree, & Rohrer, 1995), suggesting that both treatment and aftercare for older adults must address depression, loneliness, boredom, and social support.

The follow-up process assists staff in helping clients reinforce the gains made during the active treatment stage, provides opportunities for program evaluation through the use of repeated measures analyses of the assessments, permits evaluation of clients' well-being via self-reports and reports by "significant others," and provides opportunities for "touch-up" and review sessions for individuals returning for visits.

To reduce the likelihood of relapse for older adults, several criteria should be met. The follow-up program should encourage honesty in self-reporting, avoid confrontation, gradually (rather than abruptly) taper the person from attendance at the active phase of treatment, preschedule follow-up visits, include reports from family or significant others, and encourage clients to self-monitor their urges to drink and episodes of drinking by logging their behavior.

In GAP, clients returned to the program at 1, 3, 6, and 12 months for assessments, follow-up interviews, and socialization with active clients. Those unable to attend were contacted by telephone and interviewed on the same schedule. Clients continued to log their behavior, particularly on those days during which urges to drink were noted. The logs helped to define and record the conditions prior to the urge (situation, feelings, thoughts, persons present, the urge itself), what the client chose to do, and the consequences. The logs also provided information related to periods between data collection points, as well as data specific to "urge days," what the client did, and the outcome. Throughout active treatment and follow-up, clients were encouraged to be honest about their slips, and to share their experience about their slips with others in the group upon a return visit. Thus, slips were used as learning experiences, with clients rehearsing the components of the drinking behavior chain and the skills used or not used. Those in follow-up who slipped were encouraged to recontact the program and return for a day or two, and enter an appropriate group. Alternatives to return visits were detailed discussions over the phone or individual sessions. Through such methods, skills were refreshed and reasons for not using available skills were discussed.

Case Examples

In this section, we illustrate how the assessment and CBT/SM approaches are utilized in planning, delivery, and follow-up of treatment, using two case examples from our Substance Abuse Program for the Elderly. The cases illustrate how to identify each client's substance use behavior chain, plan the treatment, and teach the skills necessary to manage antecedents for drinking, recognize thoughts and self-statements which previously seemed automatic or habitual in nature, and to enhance self-control and self-efficacy in coping.

Case 1: A Passive Homemaker. Mrs. R. was a 55-year-old, Caucasian, married woman identified by a community referral network established by the program. She reported that she felt her drinking problem had begun at age 35. Her treatment history showed three hospitalizations for substance abuse in the prior 21 years, attendance at AA groups about seven years prior to admission, and treatment for depression and anxiety by a psychiatrist during the same period of time. Using the GAP-DP, we focused on the 30-day period preceding her last drink (approximately five weeks prior to admission). Many questions focus on a "typical day" of drinking during those 30 days, especially the *first* drink on a typical day. Inconsistencies are discussed during treatment. Relying on her self-report the following information was obtained:

Drinking Pattern. When asked to select a drinking pattern, she chose "Steady Drinker (drinking almost every day)" as opposed to weekend or periodic drinker, and reported having one or more drinks on 17 out of the 30 days, and being intoxicated 9 of those days. When asked to define "intoxicated," she reported that it meant "slurring words and not being organized."

Quantity Consumed. On a typical drinking day during that period, she reported drinking a pint of vodka. Note that this is inconsistent with the reported number of days intoxicated, especially since Mrs. R. was a petite woman. More alcohol was consumed on weekdays when her husband was away working. She estimated spending $75 each week on liquor, an amount of money more consistent with greater alcohol use and intoxication for a petite woman.

Drinking Behavior Chain. Table 7.1 shows Mrs. R.'s drinking behavior chain developed using her responses to sections of the GAP-DP focusing on antecedents of the first drink on a typical day of drinking and consequences experienced while drinking.

The information in the Figure actually points to two similar chains. The first, and most typical, was that Mrs. R. drank when home, alone, feeling bored about housework, after her husband left for work. While she had both positive and negative consequences right after she began drinking, she reported the most desirable thing about drinking was that "It made me able to do what I needed to do. It would relieve tension." Also, she stated "I drank because I felt inadequate, insecure, and guilty." The second chain was when Mrs. R. drank in response to her husband being around the house and "nagging" her about the housework. In that chain, she drank to get even with her husband.

Based upon the GAP-DP data, it was decided that Mrs. R.'s plan should include groups focusing on anger and frustration (assertiveness training), on problem-solving skills to identify potential solutions (e.g., scheduling her day, identifying methods for rewarding herself for doing the household chores), and on how to manage tension and anxiety. A counselor would meet with the husband or other key family members to attempt to suggest ways for the husband to respond differently. Mrs. R. was trained in self-management skills related to the issues noted above. She successfully acquired those skills (reaching established criteria), and was deemed ready for discharge by staff and Mrs. R.

Follow-Up. Each successful program "graduate" was followed up at 1, 3, 6, and 12 months. Mrs. R. did well until 8 months after discharge. At that time, according to her self-report, her husband had been "critical all weekend. I dreaded listening to him gripe." As a result, she reported feeling tense and depressed, and began drinking one day ". . . so I wouldn't have to listen to him. He gives me the silent treatment when I drink." An additional slip occurred at about 10 months post-discharge, for similar reasons. On each occasion, she consumed a half pint of vodka and became intoxicated.

Although Mrs. R. did not maintain abstinence throughout the 1-year follow-up, in comparison with her preadmission levels of drinking in which she was intoxicated about 9 out of 30 days and consuming a pint of vodka each weekday, two slips within a 1-year follow-up period are a marked improvement. The husband reported dramatic improvement in her drinking and interpersonal behavior. In addition, during a debriefing or refresher session, her recall of the antecedents to her slip (husband's nagging) demonstrated that she could identify her abusive drinking chain, which increased the potential for self-management.

Table 7.1 The Drinking Behavior Chain for Case #1

Antecedents			→	Behavior	→ Consequences	
SITUATIONS/ THOUGHTS	**FEELINGS**	**CUES**	**URGES**	**DRINK**	**IMMEDIATE/ SHORT-TERM**	**LONG-TERM**
Alone, thinking about cleaning the house, doing my chores.	Guilty about not doing my work Depressed about not giving 100% of my capabilities Lonely—there by myself	Every day as my husband went to work, he asked "Are you going to be OK?" (She felt insulted by the way he asked it) 2 p.m. Vodka in closet	"I hate it when he asks that!" "I need something to help me with my boring housework. "I hate it!"	Vodka	Strong (+) "could do housework & cope" Tense (-) "Afraid I'd get caught" Guilty (-) "Not doing my job well at home" Lonely (-) "At home, alone"	Couldn't think straight (-)
Husband "nags" me about housework not being done	Angry at my husband and at myself (for not doing my chores)	Seeing my house in a mess	"It will mask the pain for a while" "I'll show him!"	Vodka	Felt Secure (+) Relieved tension (+)	I was a burden to my family (-)

Case 2: A Veteran Who Used Alcohol and Medications. Mr. S.'s case presented a different challenge, i.e., that of an individual who abused both alcohol and prescribed medications, sometimes separately and sometimes mixing the two. As a result, we used two structured interview assessments, the GAP-DP to identify the drinking behavior chain, and a similar instrument we had developed for our program to identify the medication misuse behavior chain.

The medication "profile" addressed such issues as the types and amounts of prescribed and over-the-counter medications used, the number of prescribing physicians, any misuse of medications (overuse, discontinuing against physician advice, taking medications at wrong times or for wrong reasons, etc.), and finally, the antecedents and consequences of the misused medications (i.e., the medication misuse behavior chain).

Mr. S. was a 71-year-old, Hispanic, married man referred from the geropsychiatric unit of the local Veterans Affairs (VA) hospital. He reported a long history of alcohol abuse, beginning in his 20s after he left the military in World War II. Mr. S. had been a prisoner of war in Italy and Germany, experiencing numerous atrocities and deprivation. At admission to the SAPE program, he was receiving 100% service-connected disability benefits.

His stepfather labeled Mr. S. as having a drinking problem at age 33, but Mr. S. reported that his drinking problem had begun at age 40. He was arrested about 6 years prior to admission after mixing alcohol and medications and getting into a traffic accident. He reported four suicide attempts in the six years prior to admission and psychiatric inpatient treatment at the local VA hospital for suicidal ideation, depression, and post-traumatic stress disorder. In the year prior to admission to our program, Mr. S. was also treated for medication abuse.

Upon admission to SAPE, he reported that he was taking several prescription medications for a variety of gastrointestinal problems (ranitidine, simethicone, aluminum hydroxide gel), doxepin for his "nerves," salsalate for arthritis, and carisoprodol for back pain. In addition he consumed over-the-counter medications for pain and gastrointestinal problems, including acetaminophen and magnesium-aluminum hydroxide compounds. Responses on the Beck Depression Inventory (score = 20), Geriatric Depression Scale (score = 24), and State-Trait Anxiety Inventory (score = 41) indicated high levels of depression and anxiety for which Mr. S. expressed a desire to learn healthier ways of coping.

The following information was derived from the alcohol and medication profiles:

Drinking Pattern. Mr. S. described himself as a "periodic drinker," but reported drinking about 16 days out of the recent 30 days prior to his last drink, and being intoxicated on only five of those days. When asked to define "intoxicated" he reported it meant he "couldn't see straight." He reported this as "less" when compared with previous 30-day periods.

Quantity Consumed. In the most recent 30-day period (preceding the last drink), he reported drinking 7 ounces of Scotch on a typical day. The reported period of consumption each day (from about 3:00 P.M. until after dinner) suggests a greater frequency of intoxication. Mr. S. weighed about 165 pounds. He estimated spending $100 dollars each week on Scotch.

Medication Misuse. Mr. S. reported taking extra doxepin and carisoprodol or saving up daily doses for use at night.

Substance Use Chain. The drinking and medication use behavior chains for Mr. S. are illustrated in the Table 7.2.

The first chain usually began with him at home, feeling anxious and thinking about past experiences. At the same time he looked forward to being with his friends at the bar. Typically, he went to the bar to play pool or socialize with friends in the afternoon. At the bar, he would observe everyone drinking and having a good time, then feel like joining them and relaxing. All of his self-reported immediate/short-term consequences of that first drink were positive, relating to having a good time with friends, or feeling relaxed (not anxious). Long-term consequences were all negative, reflecting how he treated his family while intoxicated.

The second chain shown in the table is an attempt to illustrate how he misused certain of his prescribed medications (those with psychoactive effects), by focusing on when he would consume more than the prescribed amount. Sometimes this misuse occurred in combination with drinking. This medication use chain suggests both psychological and physical triggers to the misuse. Usually he was at home with his wife (situations). He would feel depressed, anxious, tense, or agitated prior to the first use of the medications (feelings). He also experienced pain in his back (and other parts of the body) which, in turn, prompted him to remember the location of his medications (cues). His medication use urges, or self-statements, again related to a need to relax and to forget his physical and financial troubles. As before, the immediate consequences were rewarding—feeling relaxed, peaceful, and pain-free. The long-term consequences of continued misuse were all negative—feeling sleepy, walking crooked, feeling guilty

Table 7.2 The Drinking Behavior Chain for Case #2

Antecedents			→	Behavior	→ Consequences	
SITUATIONS/ THOUGHTS	**FEELINGS**	**CUES**	**URGES**	**DRINK**	**IMMEDIATE/ SHORT-TERM**	**LONG-TERM**
Feeling nervous when home. Thinking about bad experiences.	Restless about being alone	After lunch—go to bar or club	"I'd like to feel relaxed"	Scotch	Friendly (+) and Happy (+) "being with my friends & drinking buddies"	Getting drunk (-) Angry at myself (-)
Go to bar to play pool with friends	Wanted to fit in with everyone	Seeing my friends drinking, having a good time	"I'd like being with my friends and drinking"	Scotch	Relaxed (+) "didn't feel nervous anymore"	The "things" I did to my wife and kids" (-)
SITUATIONS/ THOUGHTS	**FEELINGS**	**CUES**	**URGES**	**MEDICA-TIONS**	**IMMEDIATE/ SHORT-TERM**	**LONG-TERM**
At home, working around house, thinking about past Talking to wife	Depressed, nervous, tense Agitated—about how things are going	Back pain Medications in kitchen cabinet	"I want to forget my troubles" "I need to calm down" "Need to stop bad thoughts" "4 or 5 pills will be better"	Doxepin Carisoprodol	Relaxed (+) "not jumpy" Peaceful (+) "pain going away"	Get sleepy (-) and walk crooked (-) Felt guilty (-) taking too many medications and mixing them with alcohol

about mixing alcohol and medications, exacerbating physical complaints, and marital difficulties.

The treatment plan focused on "how to manage anxiety and tension" through behavioral techniques employed in a self-management group addressing that area. Mr. S. learned to identify the self-statements and thoughts associated with tension/anxiety, how to interrupt those cognitions using thought-stopping techniques, and replace the cognitions using covert assertion. Also, he learned progressive muscle relaxation as a coping mechanism for tension reduction, as well as alternatives to socializing in bars with his "drinking buddies." Thus, expanded use of community resources was instituted via involvement in social support network development. Mr. S. was also taught "drink refusal" skills (how to refuse a drink without losing a friend), as well as better communication skills when conversing with his wife. The latter was done via problem solving and role-playing groups. In summary, the training groups Mr. S. entered were directly related to the high-risk situations (antecedents and consequences) that constituted the basis of his diagrammed drinking and medication behavior chains.

During the active phase of treatment, Mr. S. experienced a slip in which he reported two mixed drinks (scotch) in response to celebrations among his friends in watching soldiers return from Operation Desert Storm in the Persian Gulf War. He reported feeling anxious and tense and didn't want to hurt his friends' feelings by refusing the celebratory drinks. However, using a combination of his drink refusal skills in combination with "relapse prevention" skills taught to all clients, Mr. S. stopped after that slip on that occasion. Another slip followed a couple of weeks later. But, it was a slip that he planned without our knowledge. He was at the wedding of his niece, and he and his wife had decided in advance that he would have a single glass of champagne, a toast to the bride and groom. He did so and stopped.

Follow-Up. During the 12-month follow-up period, Mr. S. had another two slips; one minor and one more significant. The minor slip occurred about one month after discharge and the second slip occurred about two months after discharge. Mr. S. approached the staff for clarification of the chains involved in his slips, and discussion of the relevance of his previously acquired self-management skills to the triggers in those. The slips were diagrammed and used as teaching mechanisms for the client as well as current group members. Mr. S. never returned to his pretreatment drinking levels or associated problems during the 12-month follow-up period.

Conclusions

The assessment and treatment planning approaches described in this chapter correspond well to the recommendations by the TIP expert panel (Center for Substance Abuse Treatment, 1998). The programs offered age-specific treatment, CBT/SM approaches, and avoidance of confrontation and labeling. In GAP, because confrontation was not permitted, we found that clients were often more willing to share their slips during treatment as well as during follow-up/aftercare. Clients understood that the slips would be used for instructional purposes both for themselves and other group members. The slip would be diagrammed, solutions brainstormed, and corrective behaviors role played. Clients were invited to call or visit as they felt necessary for "booster/refresher" sessions and conversations. Thus, there was an easy relationship and openness to admitting slips not customary to many alcohol treatment programs. Staff members from the GET SMART program in California have reported similar rapport with their clients.

Another aspect of the CBT/SM programs is that success is not measured simply in terms of abstinence. In GAP, recommendations for discharge were based not on roundtable discussions where clinical staff offered impressions, beliefs, hopes, etc., but were based instead upon clients' successful acquisition and implementation of skills specific to their known antecedents for alcohol abuse. Clients demonstrated this in group treatments by being able to diagram, understand, and prevent or terminate their individual drinking behavior chains, and use of the appropriate skills learned in treatment during high-risk situations experienced when not in treatment sessions. In addition, using role plays and pretest/posttest quizzes, clients demonstrated mastery of the skills taught within the groups. Through the use of techniques such as consequences cards, knowledge of hotline telephone numbers, and encouragement to recontact program staff as needed, clients were taught skills related to coping with a slip, and how to prevent that slip from becoming a relapse. Once discharge readiness was determined, a "weaning" process was scheduled. Clients were gradually tapered from the program. When needed, clients were encouraged to speak with staff and revisit treatment groups either on a "booster" or "refresher" basis as needed. For self-monitoring of drinking, clients recorded daily behavior, the presence or absence of urges to drink, and any drinking behavior during active phases of treatment and in follow-up (Dupree et al., 1984).

While few age-specific treatment programs exist, the technology for implementing an age-specific CBT/SM curriculum to prevent relapse does exist. The GET SMART program demonstrated how the curriculum and treatment methodology can be disseminated to other sites and is applicable to individuals who abuse one or more substances.

References

Center for Substance Abuse Treatment. (1998). *Substance abuse among older adults* (TIP Series, No. 26). (DHHS Publication No. SMA 98–3179). Rockville, MD: Department of Health and Human Services.

Dupree, L. W., Broskowski, H., & Schonfeld, L. (1984). The Gerontology Alcohol Project: A behavioral treatment program for elderly alcohol abusers. *Gerontologist, 24,* 510–516.

Dupree, L. W., & Schonfeld, L. (1996). Substance abuse treatment for older adults: A cognitive-behavioral and self-management approach. Manual developed for UPBEAT Project, Department of Veterans Affairs and Center for Substance Abuse Treatment.

Dupree, L. W., & Schonfeld, L. (in press). Current treatment approaches for older alcohol abusers. In E. S. L. Gomberg and R. Zucker (Editors), *Drugs and aging.* New York: Haworth Press.

Graham, K., Brett, P. J., & Baron, J. (1997). A harm reduction approach to treating older adults: The clients speak. In P. G. Erickson, D. M. Riley, Y. W. Cheung, & P. A. O'Hare (Editors). *Harm reduction: A new direction for drug policies and programs* (pp. 428–452). Toronto: University of Toronto Press.

Marlatt, G. A., & Gordon, J. R. (1985). *Relapse prevention: Maintenance strategies in the treatment of addictive behaviors.* New York: Guilford Press.

National Institute on Drug Abuse and National Institute on Alcohol Abuse and Alcoholism. (1990). *National drug and alcoholism treatment unit survey (NDATUS). 1989 Main findings report.* (DHHS Publication No. ADM 91–1729). Rockville, MD: Author.

Saunders, S., Graham, K., Flower, M., & White-Campbell, M. (1992). The COPA project as a model for the management of early dementia in the community. In G. M. M. Jones & B. M. L. Miesen (Editors), *Care-giving in dementia: Research and applications.* New York: Tavistock/Routledge.

Schonfeld, L., & Dupree, L. W. (1991). Antecedents of drinking for early-and late-onset elderly alcohol abusers. *Journal of Studies on Alcohol, 52,* 587–591.

Schonfeld, L., Dupree, L.W., Dickson-Fuhrmann, E., Royer, C., McDermott,

C., Rosansky, J. S., Taylor, S., & Jarvik, L. F. (2000). Cognitive-behavioral treatment of older veterans with substance abuse problems. *Journal of Geriatric Psychiatry and Neurology, 13,* 124–129.

Schonfeld, L., Dupree, L. W., & Rohrer, G. E. (1995). Age-related differences between younger and older alcohol abusers. *Journal of Clinical Geropsychology, 1,* 219–227.

West, P., & Graham, K. (1999). Clients speak: Participatory evaluation of a nonconfrontational addictions treatment program for older adults. *Journal of Aging and Health, 11,* 540–564.

8

Further Strategies in the Treatment of Aging Alcoholics

Roland M. Atkinson and Sahana Misra

A Menu of Treatment Options

The strategies available for intervening to help risky and problem drinkers are impressively rich and varied, as can be seen in Table 8.1. Prior chapters have presented information about a number of these treatment options, beginning with brief interventions to modify alcohol consumption, brief motivational counseling methods to overcome patients' resistence to modifying their drinking behavior, and pharmacological methods to deter drinking (see chapter 6 in this volume), and cognitive-behavioral treatment (see chapter 7 in this volume). Our purpose in this chapter is to review briefly a number of other strategies that have been employed to assist older alcoholics (see also Atkinson, Turner & Tolson, 1998).

Intervention

When brief intervention and motivational counseling do not succeed in influencing a person with heavy or problem drinking to reduce consumption

Table 8.1 Treatment Approaches for Persons With Alcohol Problems

APPROACH	INDICATIONS[a]	DISCUSSED IN CHAPTER
Brief intervention	Risky, mild prob	(Fleming's)
Motivational counseling	Risky, prob and AUDs resistent to change	(Fleming's)
Intervention	Prob, AUDs not responsive to measures above	(This chapter)
Outreach, in-home visits	Prob, AUDs unable to attend office visits	(This chapter)
Pharmacologic treatments	Prob, AUDs, patients with comorbidities	(Fleming, Atkinson & Misra's)
Cognitive-behavioral treatment	Prob, AUDs	(Schonfeld & Dupree's)
Case management	AUDs, especially those with complex problems	(This chapter)
Monitoring alcohol & drug use	Risky, prob, AUDs	(This chapter)
Group treatment	AUDs	(This chapter)
Work with collaterals	Prob, AUDs	(This chapter)
Alcoholics Anonymous	AUDs	(This chapter)
Residential treatment	Severe AUDs with uncontrolled drinking	(This chapter)
Inpatient treatment	Severe AUDs, especially with comorbidities	(This chapter)

[a]Indications: "Risky"—at risk drinkers, those consuming alcohol at high levels but without current alcohol-related problems; "Prob"—persons with current alcohol-related problems that do not meet criteria for an alcohol use disorder; "AUDs"—persons suffering from an alcohol-use disorder as defined by DSM-IV, either Alcohol Dependence or Alcohol Abuse.

or enter treatment, another approach that has often been successful is "Intervention." This method was first developed at the Johnson Institute in Minneapolis (Atkinson, 1985; Johnson, 1973; Merrill, 1990). In this approach, persons who are intimately acquainted with the patient's drinking problem first meet with a professional leader, without the patient present, to share their perceptions of the problem. Persons typically included are the spouse or other close relatives, and possibly an employer, clergyman, health professional or close friends familiar with the situation. Through discussion, each person refines the comments they intend to share with the patient at a subsequent meeting. The emphasis is placed on presenting factual observations in an emotionally supportive manner, without recrimination or negative judgment, similar to the approach used in motivational counseling. This discussion thus serves as a rehearsal for the intervention meeting itself that closely follows. At this meeting with the patient, led by the professional, each person shares with the patient his or her prepared comments on their observations and concerns about the patient's drinking and its negative consequences. The goal of intervention is for the patient to take the initial step toward alcoholism treatment.

Special care must be taken in structuring interventions with older alcoholics. Limiting the number of attendees to no more than two or three may avoid overwhelming the patient, both emotionally and cognitively. The principal caretaking relative (usually a spouse or adult child) and a primary medical provider or caseworker, for example, might constitute an adequate number. Participants need to communicate a caring attitude and respect for the patient very clearly and supportively. Including young relatives for whom the patient has been a highly respected figure is usually unwise, as the following vignette illustrates:

> Mr. Z., 66, had been resistent to entering alcoholism treatment until an intervention that included two of his grandchildren who were mid-adolescents. Interviewed four months after enrolling in an outpatient program for older alcoholics, he said, " . . . I'm glad I came into treatment. I feel better in many ways now that I'm not drinking. But, I'll tell you one thing bad. I'll never forgive you people for talking about my drinking in front of my grandchildren. I still feel ashamed whenever I see them."

Outreach Approaches

When persons suspected of suffering from serious alcohol problems refuse to seek care for drinking problems, they may still be willing to receive visits at home. In-home services have been reported from several sites (Bissell & Sweeney, 1981; Fredriksen, 1992) and particularly from the long-running Community Older Persons Alcohol (COPA) program in Toronto (Graham et al., 1995). Essential to such an approach is willingness of the staff to let clients define the problems they see as most important, and respond to these needs as a first priority. Delaying a focus on alcohol and drug misuse may be necessary if the client communicates more urgently perceived needs. Staff may also wish to influence the client to agree at some point to begin visits to the clinic, but this issue should not become a source of conflict. Some clients are more likely to remain responsive to treatment if home-based care continues on a more open-ended basis, even for months or years, as demonstrated in the COPA program.

In-home outreach efforts combine elements of brief intervention and motivational counseling with case management, the topic we will discuss next. But, to reiterate, the distinctive character of in-home outreach is related to the fact that many of the clients resist participation in clinic-based care and insist on defining their problems in their own fashion. These realities need to be respected by the caseworker, who must then make appropriate adjustments in the goals, pace, priorities, and methods of intervention.

Case Management

Individual case management is an essential component in the treatment of nearly all older individuals with alcohol dependence. For those with inadequate social support networks, and especially in the absence of a reliable community caregiver, case management can be the crucial factor to assure that treatment goals are achieved, even when other methods, such as support groups, are also used. When a particular program or practice setting does not include three or more older alcoholics (a miminum number for a peer-group approach), "one-on-one" case management may be the one best possible approach to treatment for the older patient. Case management typically occurs in the outpatient setting, although this approach can also be practiced in the long-term care residential care setting. Depending upon the setting and circumstances, the case manager might be a primary care physician or nurse practitioner, senior services caseworker, addictions counselor, or mental health professional.

Table 8.2 Roles of the Case Manager Through Stages of Treatment

Stage of Treatment	Roles of the Case Manager
Decision for Abstinence and Treatment	• Establish therapeutic alliance • Evaluate positives and negatives of drinking and entering treatment • Establish treatment plan • Establish contact with family members
Early Remission	• Establish therapeutic alliance and contact with family members (if this is the initial point of contact) • Monitor alcohol use • Educate about, and manage, relapses • Assure adherence with health care and other aspects of treatment plan • Assist with referrals for housing, financial aid, volunteer, or paid work, etc. • Assist with rebuilding social network to include nondrinking associates • Establish communications with patient's primary care physician
Drinking Relapses	• Reengage patient into treatment rapidly (outreach efforts) • Provide empathy and encouragement
Continuing Care (Aftercare)	• Monitor alcohol use • Identify and provide referrals for activities consistent with sober lifestyle • Provide assistance with other psychosocial issues, e.g., rebuilding relationships with spouse, children, and others

The case manager works toward rapidly establishing rapport—a positive therapeutic alliance—with the patient, and with family or other collaterals if available. The case manager then provides support and practical assistance to the patient, ideally throughout the entire course of treatment. A primary care-based case management model for older persons with alcohol use disorders, using nurse practitioners as case managers, has been tested at the University of Pennsylvania Treatment Research Center (Kaempf, O'Donnell, & Oslin, 1999; Volpicelli, Pettinati, McLellan, & O'Brien, 2000), with some positive effects on treatment response. Various roles of a case manager at different points in treatment are summarized in Table 8.2 and discussed next.

Decision to Enter Treatment

Sometimes the person designated to be case manager is a professional who has worked with the patient prior to the decision to enter treatment for alcoholism. At this stage the case manager can provide valuable assistance to the patient in weighing the pros and cons of the drinking behavior. A review of alcohol-related medical, mental health and social problems, and abnormal laboratory test results (e.g., abnormal liver function) should be conducted. Once the decision to enter treatment has been made, a treatment plan is established. Although this plan may be made by others, the case manager will be in a pivotal position to arrange appropriate referrals and thus requires knowledge of available community treatment resources.

Early Remission (Early Recovery)

More commonly, a case manager is chosen after treatment has begun. During the early weeks and months of recovery, the case manager focuses on helping the patient to identify triggers for drinking relapse. The patient is also helped to resist the impulsive tendency to drink rather than attempt alternative coping strategies. Another often pivotal role is in arranging for planned follow-up evaluations, consultations, and information sharing, particularly in cases that are medically or psychiatrically complex, or that require services delivered by multiple providers (see chapter 9 in this volume). All too often, without a case manager watching over all intended steps in the treatment plan, such follow-ups may not occur and the patient becomes "lost between the cracks" in the health care system. When patients have been taking prescription benzodiazepines or opioids in conjunction with alcohol abuse, it is wise to contact the prescribing physician early in treatment and continue to involve this physician in treatment planning, especially in continuing care. All too often the substance abuse treatment program merely sends a treatment or discharge summary (or worse, none at all) to a physician with whom the treatment team or case manager has had no contact. Also at this early point, many patients clearly face for the first time the need to resolve financial and housing problems. The case manager should be familiar with local housing options that will help sustain a sober lifestyle, e.g., alcohol-free group homes. Important activities may include arranging linkages to career counseling or vocational rehabilitation programs for persons capable of rejoining the work force, facilitating the patient's application for Social Security, Medicare, or other health insurance or disability benefits, and perhaps helping to arrange for a primary health care provider.

Anticipating and Responding to Drinking Relapses

Since drinking lapses are common in the course of recovery from alcohol dependence, the case manager should anticipate and discuss this possibility with the patient early in treatment. Early discussion, before such drinking lapses occur, is highly useful for several reasons. First, newly recovering patients often think that relapse is not a possibility, and may react with unjustified or excessive pessimism and demoralization following a lapse unless prepared for this. And it is important for the case manager to establish a trusting and respectful rapport that will make possible both routine monitoring of possible drinking (see next section) as well as candid, nonjudgmental discussion of drinking lapses when they do occur. The patient needs to realize that it is not the case manager's goal to respond punitively if relapse occurs. Instead patient and case manager should jointly plan for responses that they should make, i.e., special steps to be taken, in the event of relapse. Because some patients tend to react after relapse by avoiding contact or dropping out of treatment, outreach efforts may be required, such as phone calls or home visits after missed appointments to help the patient successfully reengage in treatment.

Continuing Care (Aftercare)

Individual case management is often required beyond the acute phase of treatment. As many elders reach the end of active treatment, the transition from relying on the treatment program to relying on community resources for support may seem a daunting task, despite efforts to anticipate this transition. This is especially true for patients whose social circle before treatment consisted primarily of drinking partners or tavern life. The case manager can guide the patient to rediscover old pastimes or consider alternative social outlets and activities, and thus needs to be aware of nearby senior centers, clubs, gyms, and so on. Referral to a recreational therapist may be in order, as may further career counseling or guidance on appropriate settings for contributing as volunteer workers. The case manager can also encourage the patient to remain linked to the program through an "alumni group" or through informal socializing with other former patients who have become valued acquaintances. Finally, this point of stabilized sobriety may be the first time when conditions are right for the patient to attempt to reconnect with alienated family members. The case manager can facilitate these efforts or refer the patient to a family therapist for such assistance.

Monitoring of Alcohol and Drug Use

Monitoring of alcohol and drug use is not only useful as a means of gauging progress in reducing consumption but can be a powerful intervention in itself. Maintaining a daily diary of alcohol consumption, for example, can aid a risky drinker in both documenting and reducing alcohol intake in response to brief intervention efforts. Staff monitoring of substance use in recovering outpatient older problem drinkers is desirable. Such monitoring should be conducted in the spirit of assisting rather than intruding. One should query patients at clinic appointments about alcohol use since the last contact. In a group-based treatment program, asking about alcohol use *in the group* makes open discussion of recent alcohol use a "normative" activity that is "everybody's business," just like management of life problems and difficulties in relationships. Ongoing efforts to obtain information from collaterals (spouse, other cohabitants, caregivers) about the patient's drinking is also useful.

Performance of random, unannounced breath and urine examinations for alcohol and potentially abusable drugs is also desirable. Such checks cannot, of course, be expected to catch many instances of drinking relapse or surreptitious psychoactive drug use. Instead this testing is practiced primarily because of the strong "message" conveyed to patients that the staff are striving to be conscientious in their monitoring efforts, as we desire the clients themselves to be. Random urine testing can also yield useful and sometimes surprising information. For example, our colleagues, Kania and Kofoed (1984), found that nearly 10% of patients in our older adult outpatient alcoholism treatment program had urine screening tests that were "positive" for the presence of unsuspected benzodiazepines, a class of prescribed sedative-hypnotic medications with high dependence potential that these patients had agreed not to use without first discussing the matter with program staff. Such a discovery might result in useful actions. For example, a discussion with the prescribing physician about the pros and cons of continued use of such medications might be helpful.

Information from all of these sources can be used effectively by the case manager or primary counselor to assist patients in further efforts to find suitable alternative responses to life problems, other than drinking, provided that the attitude of the counselor remains respectful, positive, supportive, and nonjudgmental.

Group Treatment

Group work in the rehabilitation of older alcoholics draws on several traditions and principles (Doroff, 1977). The founders of the Fellowship of Alcoholics Anonymous (AA) in the 1930s were convinced that affiliation with a group of recovering peers was essential to success in overcoming alcoholism. The AA group could provide a social network for emotional support and affirmation of members, a resource for intervention to prevent or contain relapses and related life crises, guidance for achieving the various steps, and successful models of recovery. The seminal influence of AA helped inspire the development of group treatment in alcoholism clinics that began in the 1940s, although the success and relatively low-cost of group therapies in mental health and other settings also played a major role. Group psychotherapy has been shown to be useful in the treatment of older adults with mental disorders (Finkel, 1990).

Age-peer socialization and discussion groups were first introduced in the rehabilitation of older persons with alcoholism by Zimberg (1974), and shortly thereafter in the first National Institute on Alcohol Abuse and Alcoholism (NIAAA) demonstration project on treatment of older alcoholics (Dunlop, Skorney, & Hamilton, 1982). For aging alcoholics, a group of recovering age-mates offers peer social bonding that increases the likelihood of patients remaining engaged in treatment (Kofoed, Tolson, Atkinson, Toth, & Turner, 1987), helps fill a social void in each other's lives, serves as a stimulus for constructive and esteem-enhancing reminiscence or "life review" (Butler, 1963), and provides encouragement of each other's efforts not to drink.

The nature and methods of groups vary (Doroff, 1977). Socialization groups may focus only on camaraderie and emphasize casual conversa-

Table 8.3 Topics for "Classes" for Older Alcoholics (1998–1999, "Class of '45" Geriatric Alcoholism Clinic, Portland, Oregon, VA Medical Center)

Proposed Topic	Importance[a]
Healthy aging—how to age "successfully"	21
Coping with low moods and depression	19
Acceptance (e.g., the past, handicaps)	18
Information on community services, social security, bus systems, veterans benefits, etc.	16
Nutrition, meal preparation, healthy eating habits	16
Managing anger and resentment	15
Spirituality in the second half of life	15
Sleep problems and sleep hygiene	14
Social networks—how to connect with others	14
Death in your life—your own, family, friends	14
The search for and secret of "happiness"	14
Additional ideas for relapse prevention	13
Holiday blues	13
Over-the-counter medicines	13
Preparing "living wills" and "advance directives"	12
What to do? Structuring your free time	12
Sharing life experiences	11
Weight loss and weight management	10
Living with chronic illness and pain	10
Financial planning	9
The 12 Steps of AA and your life	6

[a]Before the series was planned, 32 active patients were asked to vote for the topics (from a prepared list) they wanted to have included in the series. The number of patients voting for each topic is listed. Most voters (31 men and 1 woman) were over age 60.

tion and events like potlucks or outings. More formal group therapy may be oriented toward, for example, emotional support, practical problem solving, resolution of interpersonal conflicts, and, of course, relapse prevention and checking (Kofoed, Tolson, Atkinson, Turner, & Toth, 1984). The group setting has been used, among other purposes, for applying cognitive-behavioral methods (Dupree, Broskowski, & Schonfeld, 1984), for counseling of several married couples concurrently, and for didactic educational offerings and structured discussions. Table 8.3 lists topics for monthly "classes," recently conducted in our outpatient program for older alcoholics. The range of topics and their relative popularity offers useful insights about the themes that older alcoholics themselves rate as important for them to learn more about.

Group treatment may not be well tolerated by persons suffering from schizophrenia or social phobia, who are best managed on a one-to-one basis by a case manager or other professional caregiver. Home visits by a public health nurse can facilitate such individual care.

Casework With Collaterals

It is axiomatic in the treatment of younger adults with alcohol use disorders that engagement of the patient's spouse or other key collaterals in the treatment process increases the likelihood of program adherence and successful outcome (Steinglass, 1977). Our group demonstrated that among older married alcoholic men who entered outpatient treatment in a special program for seniors, when spouses participated, the rate of one-year treatment completion by their husbands was over twice as high as for men whose wives did not participate (Atkinson, Tolson, & Turner, 1993; Atkinson et al., 1998).

Because older alcoholics are more likely to have become widowed or divorced by the time they enter treatment, engagement of caregiving adult children in the treatment process may be important (Dunlop et al., 1982). The work has several aspects depending upon the needs of the patient, the relative, and the relationship between them. Dealing with old resentments and alienation may be necessary to help reconstruct a loving and useful relationship. Some elders will need significant assistance, for example, with transportation, shopping, meals, arranging appointments, finding a primary care doctor or attorney, and the family member can be guided to help the patient solve these practical problems. Adult children may need education about their parent's illness, treatment, and other needs, and may need help to identify and seek assistance for their own difficulties (for example, depression and alcohol problems are not uncommon in caregiving adult childen).

Often enough, older alcoholics may have burned their bridges with their children, becoming irreparably alienated because of the damage wrought by their alcoholism over many years. In such instances one must take a broader view to assure that some influential person in a patient's social network is not overlooked but instead becomes engaged in the treatment process. Here is an example:

> Mr. H., age 56, was evaluated during his 30-day stay in a residential alcoholism treatment program. The staff noted that he had no spouse or

adult children living in the area, and thus it was assumed that no work with collaterals was possible. But Mr. H. disclosed later, after discharge and upon more careful interviewing in the outpatient program, that a nephew, himself a former heavy drinker who had been treated previously in the same program, was currently living across the street from the hospital! Nearly 2 months' time was lost before the nephew was finally contacted.

Unfortunately patients at times may not permit staff to contact collaterals, for a variety of reasons, as illustrated next.

Mr. R., age 56, referred himself for alcoholism treatment because of rapidly increasing consumption to over 30 drinks a day. Although he was motivated for treatment, the staff became concerned about the influence of his roommate, a man age 76 with whom he had lived for the past 8 years and on whom he had become financially dependent. This concern was based on the patient's report that his roommate was also a heavy daily drinker who probably needed treatment himself. Mr. R. had no relatives in the area. His roommate clearly was a key individual to attempt to engage, for the patient's sake and for his own well-being. But Mr. R. steadfastly refused to permit any staff interaction with his roommate, fearing that this man might take offense and "throw me out."

Some elderly alcoholics have outlived all known kin and are socially isolated. Nevertheless, there is often some key individual, an informal caregiver, who might be able to assist. A none too rare situation is described next.

Mr. Z., an 81-year-old widower and retired stockbroker, was rapidly deteriorating because of his heavy drinking. He had survived all known relatives, so that his affairs were overseen by the trust department of a local bank, where he had a sizable account, although Mr. Z. was still considered competent and managed his own money. Indeed, it was the trust officer assigned to his account that contacted a social worker in private practice who specializes in casework with the elderly, to seek her help. The trust officer had noted on recent visits to Mr. Z.'s apartment that the place was increasingly littered, with many empty and partially filled liquor and mixer bottles in evidence, and that Mr. Z. himself seemed more disheveled and was increasingly unable to balance his books. Through the joint efforts of the trust officer and social worker, a guardianship and medical care were arranged for Mr. Z.

AA and Other Peer-Help Strategies

There are no systematic studies of the usefulness of Alcoholics Anonymous (AA) for older persons with alcohol use disorders. What do older alcoholics say about their AA experiences? Here are the voices of several we have interviewed over the years.

Mr. B., age 61, a gregarious man, seemed to fit well into all recommended treatments. "I thought my stay in the RTP [residential treatment program] was very useful, and I also like the "Class of '45" [a special outpatient program for aging alcoholics]. But I also like to go to the AA meetings a lot. I'm attending five different [mixed-age] meetings a week right now."

Mr. C., age 69, said that "they found me at home in a coma from drinking five years ago and put me in the hospital. I've had some trouble with depression since then, but I've been going to my [mixed-age] AA meetings faithfully for the last five years and I haven't had a drop to drink."

Mr. B., age 66, after enrolling in an outpatient program for older problem drinkers, followed the program expectation that he also attend AA meetings. He began regular attendance in both mixed-age and elder-specific meetings and says "I like both the meetings I go to, they both feel comfortable and help me stay sober."

Mr. A., age 65, reminiscing about his first contact with [mixed-age] AA, at age 57, put it this way: " . . . we folks got to run things in AA rather than be bossed around by counselors. I liked that then and I still do."

Mr. R., age 60, refused to continue [mixed-age] AA participation that had been recommended by his counselor " . . . because I just can't stand to hear people swearing all the time."

Mr. R., age 71, tried attending mixed-age AA meetings at his group therapy counselor's urging, but quit after a few meetings and refused to go back. When asked to explain, he said, "It's the vulgarity. I'm offended by it. Mainly this one young woman who told how she would sleep around with lots of men to get alcohol and drugs. Hearing about that bothered me so much I couldn't sleep at night for thinking about it." When asked why, he replied, "I don't know. I just worried about her. And it [her behavior] offended me." Encouraged to try an AA meeting just for alcoholic seniors, he reported that " . . . it's much better. I feel like I'm with people like myself. I'm much more comfortable."

Mr. B., age 71, began attending an elder-specific AA chapter after suffering from a bleeding peptic ulcer and was able to stop his heavy drinking. He fit in well and did not drink for several months. For years he had also suffered from symptoms of depression, which grew worse each autumn. He said that " . . . when fall came around, I started thinking about my wife and my father and got to feeling low, and I just couldn't go to the meetings." He dropped out but did seek treatment at a special outpatient program for older alcoholic military veterans, where his depression was also diagnosed and treated.

In the absence of systematic studies, our views about AA are shaped by stories such as these. For many older problem drinkers, mixed-age AA participation may be the single best strategy to assure long-term sobriety, or at least it may be one powerful approach to be used together with others such as case management and individual counseling. For a sizable group, however, the likelihood of successful engagement in AA may hinge on the availability of meetings specially organized for older alcoholics, especially those that exclude younger polysubstance abusers. Finding conveniently located daytime meetings can be difficult for elders who do not drive or go out at night. AA is not likely to be effective as a sole strategy for sustaining sobriety in persons with significant comorbid depression or other mental disorders, unless the patient is simultaneously engaged in psychiatric treatment, and for patients with schizophrenia or social phobia AA may not be at all well tolerated. Even in mixed-age AA chapters, it is desirable for a newly entering older person to be matched with a sponsor (a person long experienced in AA who has achieved stable sobriety) who is an age-mate.

Peer assistance can take other important forms, although, like AA, these have not been systematically studied. Volunteers can be used to lead an "alumni" group—an informal socialization group for patients who have completed formal treatment. Joseph (1995) has also employed aging peer counselors, who are carefully screened, trained and supervised, to assist in engaging older nursing home patients who report recent drinking problems, to help promote morale and encourage sobriety.

Residential and Inpatient Treatment

There are circumstances where an individual may require a more intensive treatment environment than the outpatient setting can provide. Acute inpatient hospitalization may be necessary to treat the complications of prolonged heavy drinking, like gastrointestinal hemorrhage or severe depression. A period of residential treatment may be the best response if serious drinking relapses continue to punctuate attempts at outpatient treatment. The American Society of Addiction Medicine (ASAM) has developed guidelines to assist clinicians in matching patients to the most appropriate treatment setting. The ASAM Patient Placement Criteria include several biopsychosocial dimensions, and a particular patient's current status on these dimensions can indicate the best setting for optimal care (ASAM, 1996). These dimensions include (1) the potential for serious alcohol withdrawal symptoms; (2) biomedical conditions and complication; (3) emotional and behavioral conditions and complications; (4) treatment resistence; and (5) optimal recovery environment. Levels of service in the ASAM approach range from outpatient to medically managed intensive inpatient services. Another helpful guide to determining the appropriate treatment setting is the American Psychiatric Association's (APA) Practice Guidelines for the Treatment of Patients With Substance Abuse Disorders. Indications for residential and inpatient treatment are summarized in Table 8.4 and discussed next, based on guidance from both the ASAM and APA perspectives.

Table 8.4 Indications for Residential and Inpatient Treatment of Persons With Alcohol Use Disorders

Residential treatment:	
	• Pattern of high-volume daily drinking or prolonged binges (days, weeks)
	• Inability to cease drinking
	• Proximity of drinking partners and locales
	• Lack of nondrinking social support network
	• Marginal "readiness" for treatment
	• Impulsive behavior pattern
Inpatient treatment:	
	Detoxification:
	• Prior episodes of complicated withdrawal from alcohol (e.g., delirium, seizures)
	• Comorbid medical disorder that could worsen during withdrawal from alcohol (e.g., cardiovascular, diabetes mellitus)
	Acute treatment needed for other conditions:
	• Comorbid medical disorder (e.g., cardiac, liver, gastrointestinal)
	• Comorbid psychiatric disorder (e.g., suicide risk, depression, psychosis)

Note. From APA (1995) and ASAM (1996) guidelines. Adapted with permission.

Inpatient Treatment

Costly care on acute hospital units is most commonly utilized for medically or psychiatrically "high-risk" patients. During detoxification, aging alcohol dependent persons are likely to have more severe withdrawal symptoms than younger patients and to require larger sedative doses to control these symptoms (Brower, Mudd, Blow, Young, & Hill, 1994; Liskow, Rinck, Campbell, & DeSouza, 1989). Thus clinicians should consider inpatient detoxification for older patients who have recently been drinking at high daily-dose levels, especially those who have a prior history of major withdrawal symptoms, such as delirium tremens or seizures. Older patients who have comorbid medical problems should probably also be detoxified in an inpatient setting. Examples are patients with difficult-to-control diabetes mellitus or severe cardiovascular disorders. Acute, life-threatening complications of alcoholism, like gastrointestinal hemorrhage, severe liver disease, severe major depression, or alcohol-induced psychosis, require that initial care occur on an acute medical or psychiatric inpatient unit. Another reason for inpatient treatment is repeated failed attempts at outpatient treatment because of resistence to care or poor impulse control, when continued drinking is causing significant impairment of medical or psychiatric status.

Residential Alcoholism Treatment

Some patients may require care, for up to several weeks, in a longer-term residential treatment setting as part of their treatment plan, either at the beginning of care or during a serious drinking relapse. A residential care program may or may not be attached to a medical center, but in either case a patient entering residential treatment should not be suffering from an acute medical or psychiatric disorder that requires acute inpatient care. Treatment is often under the direct supervision of nonmedical personnel, although consulting physicians in medicine and psychiatry are available. The fundamental indication for residential treatment is a judgment based on thorough assessment that the alcohol-dependent individual at the moment will not be able to sustain sobriety without this approach. Persistent heavy drinking despite outpatient intervention and treatment efforts is the major feature for persons requiring this service. One consideration is the status and nature of the patient's primary social support network. As mentioned elsewhere, many alcoholic patients have alienated family and friends, and their remaining associations often are with persons who themselves are problem drinkers. Another issue to weigh is the patient's current community living arrangement. Alcohol or illicit drugs may be more accessible around inner-city, single-room occupancy hotels. Some patients find that their favorite nearby tavern is irresistible. Residential treatment can temporarily break the cycle of daily drinking and buy time for arranging more stable alternative housing and social supports. When treatment readiness is marginal, resistence runs high or the patient suffers from poor impulse control, residential treatment may offer temporary external structure to help the patient to initially establish sobriety.

There are some potential pitfalls and disadvantages to residential treatment for older adults. In nearly every community there are not enough older patients in need of residential treatment to sustain a program designed exclusively for this age group. Some elderly are not comfortable living in close quarters and participating in groups with younger alcoholics. Staff on mixed-age units may lack sufficient knowledge to monitor medical status and adjust activity demands accordingly. Some of these problems are illustrated in the following section.

Patient Responses to Residential Treatment

As with AA, older persons vary in their reaction to mixed-age residential treatment. Here are some comments by men admitted to a veterans hospital, mixed-age, 30-day residential treatment program run along somewhat rigid, "tough love" lines.

> Mr. E., age 60, said that residential treatment " . . . was very useful, it was rigid, like the Army, which I also liked. I learned a lot. I found I was living behind a wall I didn't know was there."

> Mr. G., age 59, said residential treatment " . . . was too stressful, intense, demanding, depressing. I was offended by the staff's use of profanity." He negotiated discharge after 2 days.

> Mr. K., age 64, said that on the unit " . . . I felt isolated the first 4 days, but then progressively got more involved. I think it was a real positive experience."

As mentioned before, a danger in a mixed-age program is that the special needs and limitations of older patients may not be properly addressed. Here are two examples:

Mr. H., age 56, had trouble relating to younger men on the unit with multiple drug use and serious social problems. He also couldn't hear comments in group meetings over half the time. He much preferred an outpatient group treatment program for seniors.

Mr. T., age 65, developed chest pain on his 11th day on the unit. He required medical observation for two days, and it was felt he had had an attack of angina related to participation in the exercise program required for all patients.

Alternatives to Residential Treatment

Rehabilitation-oriented skilled nursing homes or assisted living facilities are potentially excellent alternatives to mixed-age residential treatment units as more supportive settings for interdicting severe problem drinking in older adults with significant medical or psychiatric comorbidities, especially those who have cognitive impairment and special sensory limitations (Joseph, 1995). These facilities, however, may lack alcoholism-oriented case management or support groups, so that ideally the patient placed in such a facility should also be concurrently affiliated with an outpatient alcoholism treatment program.

Desired Staff Qualities

For staff providing any treatment approach—case management or group treatment, inpatient or outpatient— there are certain qualities and skills that are useful, even critical, to successful work with aging alcoholics. A keen interest in, and respect for, aging persons ranks first. This starts with such basics as honoring the amenities (Gordon, 1990). Older people typically prefer to be addressed as "Mrs. Jones" or "Mr. Smith," not as "Melba" or "Johnnie." If this basic interest is bolstered by special training in social gerontology, geriatric mental health, or geriatric health care, so much the better. Next most important is comfort in moving along slowly to accomplish treatment objectives (Gordon, 1990). This applies to the pacing of individual discussion or counseling sessions, for a slow pace and repetition are often essential if the aging patient is to properly assimilate information, answer questions or solve problems. Third is a willingness to forgo many of the tactics often employed by alcoholism treatment counselors with younger clients.

Among those techniques that older people dislike are vigorous confrontation, profanity, psychologizing, and provocation of strong emotional display, especially in group settings. These "psychojudo" tactics have little place in treating older clients, who instead benefit from emotionally supportive methods, good manners, patience, indirection, and obliqueness, especially about emotionally painful or potentially embarrassing or shameful issues, including often alcohol use. This is not to say that such matters can or should be avoided, rather that sensitivity, discretion, and a sense of appropriate timing must guide the discussions. For further discussion of staffing issues and qualifications, see the recently published best practice guidelines from the federal Center for Substance Abuse Treatment (1998). For further demonstrations of a respectful, client-centered approach tailored to the older person, see also the chapter by Gordon (1990) and the longer report from Toronto's COPA program (Graham et al., 1995).

Summary

This chapter has attempted to present a brief inventory of various services and approaches for aging alcoholics, many of which share interconnected themes such as the importance of supportive, nonjudgmental staff attitudes and the need to treat aging problem drinkers in a context that considers the full range of their health and social circumstances. This implies more intensive and costly care in some cases than brief intervention and pharmacological approaches alone would entail, as well as a high level of staff awareness about addictions, mental health problems, and social gerontology. Options and solutions for drinking problems will vary not only depending on the severity and complexity of patients' problems but also according to the community and personal resources available to patients and their families.

References

American Psychiatric Association. (1995). Practice guideline for the treatment of patients with substance use disorders: Alcohol, cocaine, opioids. *American Journal of Psychiatry, 152*(11, Suppl.).

American Society of Addiction Medicine. (1996). *Patient placement criteria for the treatment of substance-related disorders, second edition (ASAM PPC-2).* Chevy Chase, MD: American Society of Addiction Medicine.

Atkinson, R. M. (1985). Persuading alcoholic patients to seek treatment. *Comprehensive Therapy, 11*(11), 16–24.

Atkinson, R. M., Tolson, R. L., & Turner, J. A. (1993). Factors affecting outpatient treatment compliance of older male problem drinkers. *Journal of Studies on Alcohol, 54,* 102–106.

Atkinson, R. M., Turner, J. A., & Tolson, R. L. (1998). Treatment of older adult problem drinkers: Lessons learned from the "Class of '45." *Journal of Mental Health and Aging, 4,* 197–214.

Bissell, L., & Sweeney, G. (1981). Alcoholism outreach in single-room occupancies. *American Journal of Drug and Alcohol Abuse, 8,* 215–224.

Brower, K. J., Mudd, S., Blow, F. C., Young, J. P., & Hill, E. M. (1994). Severity and treatment of alcohol withdrawal in elderly versus younger patients. *Alcoholism: Clinical and Experimental Research, 18,* 196–201.

Butler, R. N. (1963). The life review: An interpretation of reminiscence in the aged. *Psychiatry, 26,* 65–76.

Center for Substance Abuse Treatment. (1998). *Substance abuse among older adults.* Treatment Improvement Protocol (TIP) Series. No. 26. USDHHS, PHS, SAMHSA, CSAT (DHHS Publication No. SMA98-3179). Rockville, MD. (A copy of this guide may be obtained at no charge by calling the National Clearinghouse for Alcohol and Drug Information at 1–800–729–6686).

Doroff, D. R. (1977). Group psychotherapy in alcoholism. In B. Kissin, & H. Begleiter (Editors), *The biology of alcoholism. Vol. 5: Treatment and rehabilitation of the chronic alcoholic* (pp. 235–258). New York: Plenum.

Dunlop, J., Skorney, B., & Hamilton, J. (1982). Group treatment for elderly alcoholics and their families. *Social Work in Groups, 5,* 87–92.

Dupree, L. W., Broskowski, H., & Schonfeld, L. (1984). The Gerontology Alcohol Project: A behavioral treatment program for elderly alcohol abusers. *The Gerontologist, 24,* 510–516.

Finkel, S. I. (1990). Group psychotherapy with older people. *Hospital and Community Psychiatry, 41,* 1189–1191.

Fredriksen, K. I. (1992). North of Market: Older women's alcohol outreach program. *The Gerontologist, 32,* 270–272.

Gordon, M. (1990). Treatment. In M. Merrill, P. G. Kraft, M. Gordon, M. M. Holmes, & B. Walker, *Chemically dependent older adults: How do we treat them?* (pp. 39–66). Center City, MN: Hazelden.

Graham, K., Saunders, S. J., Flower, M. C., Timney, C. B., White-Campbell, M., & Pietropaolo, A. Z. (1995). *Addictions treatment for older adults: Evaluation of an innovative client-centered approach.* New York: Haworth.

Johnson, V. E. (1973). *I'll quit tomorrow.* New York: Harper and Row.

Joseph, C. L. (1995). Alcohol and drug misuse in the nursing home. *The International Journal of the Addictions, 30,* 1953–1984.

Kaempf, G., O'Donnell, C., & Oslin, D. W. (1999). The BRENDA model: A psychosocial addiction model to identify and treat alcohol disorders in elders. *Geriatric Nursing, 20,* 302–304.

Kania, J., & Kofoed, L. (1984). Drug use by alcoholics in outpatient treatment. *American Journal of Drug and Alcohol Abuse, 10,* 529–534.

Kofoed, L. L., Tolson, R. L., Atkinson, R. M., Toth, R. F., & Turner, J. A. (1987). Treatment compliance of older alcoholics: An elder-specific approach is superior to "mainstreaming." *Journal of Studies on Alcohol, 48,* 47–51; correction (1987) 48, 183.

Kofoed, L. L., Tolson, R. L., Atkinson, R. M., Turner, J. A., and Toth, R. F. (1984). Elderly groups in an alcoholism clinic. In R. M. Atkinson (Editor), *Alcohol and drug abuse in old age* (pp. 35–48). Washington, DC: American Psychiatric Press.

Liskow, B. I., Rinck, C., Campbell, J., & DeSouza, C. (1989). Alcohol withdrawal in the elderly. *Journal of Studies on Alcohol, 50,* 414–421.

Merrill, M. (1990). Intervention. In M. Merrill, P. G. Kraft, M. Gordon, M. M. Holmes, & B. Walker, *Chemically dependent older adults: How do we treat them?* (pp. 1–13). Center City, MN: Hazelden.

Steinglass, P. (1977). Family therapy in alcoholism. In B. Kissin, & H. Begleiter (Editors), *The biology of alcoholism. Vol. 5: Treatment and rehabilitation of the chronic alcoholic* (pp. 259–299). New York: Plenum.

Volpicelli, J. R., Pettinati, H. M., McLellan, A. T., & O'Brien, C. P. (2000). *Enhanced medication and treatment adherence for addiction treatment: The BRENDA model.* New York: Guilford Press.

Zimberg, S. (1974). The elderly alcoholic. *Gerontologist, 14,* 221–224.

PART III

Other Addictive Problems

9

Prescription Drug Misuse: Treatment Strategies

Richard E. Finlayson and Virginia E. Hofmann

Introduction

The term "drug abuse" typically conjures up images of street people injecting themselves with powerful drugs or committing serious crimes to maintain their "habit." The term might also suggest the use of cocaine or heroin by persons of all social classes in order to make their lives more exciting. Sometimes the public resists using the term "drug abuse." Our society has grudgingly come to accept tobacco (nicotine) as a "drug," but one still hears the term "habit" used rather than the more appropriate terms "drug abuse" or "addiction."

To date our societal denial and ignorance have largely kept the topic of prescription drug misuse in the background of public discussion except for unjustified prescribing by health professionals leading to harm in their patients. For the benefit of the reader, the authors intend the term "misuse" to encompass a range or spectrum of practices and motives. These include inappropriate use arising from a lack of understanding of the drug and its purpose and effects, intentional abuse that has adverse consequences, and drug dependence. The latter is a state in which the person has developed a pattern of use characterized by psychological dependence and compulsive behavior, i.e., loss of control of the use. We also intend the term "misuse" to include inappropriate prescribing by health professionals. Finlayson (1997) has provided a general review of the topic of misuse of prescription drugs in the elderly population that can serve as background for this chapter, in which the primary focus will be on the practical management of such cases.

A Rationale for Treatment

One might ask the question, "Is this a problem which is deserving of substance abuse treatment?" The elderly do after all have more sleep problems and chronic pain, and therefore more need for sedatives and analgesics. Psychoactive substance use may, however, add to the morbidity experienced by the elderly due to their physical disorders. As an example, in a study by Ried, Johnson, and Gettman (1998), reviewing functional status of elderly patients, age and medical condition were the most significant predictors of functional status. Persons in the study receiving a benzodiazepine scored *lower* on the functional status measures, and benzodiazepine use was associated with dysfunctional status to the same extent caused by several chronic medical conditions. This effect persisted after controlling for sociodemographic characteristics and medical conditions. Stated differently, benzodiazepines had an *independent* negative effect on the functional status of these elderly. This study provides a rationale for addressing problems of misuse, abuse and dependence involving prescription drugs.

It might be argued that the problem of substance-related disorders is so uncommon in the elderly that the topic is not deserving of much attention. It is true that little attention has been paid to the problem using addiction science methodology. Most of the papers the authors are familiar with have dealt with the patterns of use of prescription drugs, their side effects in the elderly, etc. There are some reported data, primarily from clinical populations, about the prevalence of substance-related disorders. A study from the state of Virginia reported by Holroyd and Duryee (1997) provided prevalence data from a geriatric psychiatry outpatient clinic. The overall prevalence for any substance use disorder was 20%. The prevalence of benzodiazepine dependence was 11.4%; alcohol dependence was 8.6%; and prescription narcotic dependence was 1.4%. These are significant findings suggesting that in the elderly psychiatric population substance-related problems are quite common.

Mental illness in late life is a risk factor for substance abuse according to a study reported from the Mayo Clinic by Finlayson and Davis

(1994). The histories of one hundred elderly persons diagnosed as having dependence on prescription drugs were studied. General *medical factors and life stress did not correlate positively with having a drug dependence* disorder. Being female and having a mental illness diagnosis *did* correlate positively with having a drug dependence disorder, usually on benzodiazepines or opioids. Depressive disorders may present in the elderly as insomnia and chronic pain, and remain largely unrecognized, leading to prescription of the wrong medications. Thus, although we lack adequate data concerning the incidence and prevalence of drug dependence from the community dwelling elderly, we have evidence that these problems are quite common in psychiatric clinics for the elderly. Clinicians who confront mental health problems in the older population should be aware of the problem of potential misuse of psychoactive prescription drugs.

Special attention to prescription drug misuse in the elderly is also justified because of studies that reveal prescribing patterns that may be harmful to patients. To give an example, there is evidence that depression is commonly misdiagnosed in older persons and treated with benzodiazepines, rather than antidepressants (Finlayson & Davis, 1994; North, McAvoy, & Powell, 1992). Physician behavior with respect to prescribing drugs has been a topic in national conferences sponsored by the American Medical Association and in various studies and reviews in the medical literature (Hasday & Karch, 1981; Shorr, Bauwens & Landefeld, 1990; and Wesson & Smith, 1990). It has been suggested that physicians should take more responsibility for how their prescribing behavior complicates the lifestyle of their patients, and that the physician and patient share responsibility for the proper use of prescription drugs.

Barriers to Treatment

The misuse of prescription drugs may be difficult to distinguish from normal use, particularly in the elderly, for a number for reasons. Many times, the misuse is unrecognized until a problem arises, for example, falls, adverse mood changes, cognitive decline, incontinence, poor hygiene, or sleep disorders. Even when these problems are evident, it is not always recognized that the patient's use or misuse of prescription drugs is a factor. The two factors usually considered first in explaining psychosocial and physical decline are normal aging and chronic illness. Too often there is a tendency by many to assume that age *per se* is the cause of decline. In the past, for example, it was common to explain "senility" on the basis of advancing age. We now use the term "dementia" to explain such cognitive decline and know that it is a disease and not due simply to aging. Chronic illness is the usual cause of symptoms such as poor appetite, insomnia, fatigue, pain, serious cognitive decline, and depressed mood.

Assumptions that the elderly patient's symptoms are only related to aging or chronic illness can create a barrier to proper diagnosis and treatment of drug misuse. The high rates of comorbidity and overlapping symptoms often create a baffling diagnostic puzzle. The side effects of steady dosing with psychoactive substances and especially excessive use may include depression, heightened anxiety, fatigue or cognitive impairment, the very symptoms commonly associated with general medical and mental disorders. Sometimes it is not until inappropriate drug use has been reduced or eliminated that the extent of adverse effects becomes known.

Social factors may delay or prevent referral for therapy. One obstacle to recognizing self-induced drug problems is the difficulty we have in viewing an elderly patient as a "drug abuser," a term often used pejoratively. However, the continued misuse of drugs resulting in negative consequences is a criterion for drug abuse (American Psychiatric Association, 1994). Given that the elderly usually obtain the drugs within the context of a legitimate physician-patient relationship, critical examination of the drug-using behavior seems less likely to occur. The parties involved may be reluctant to admit that the patient is dependent upon a prescription drug because of the stigma of having such a problem for a patient and the negative reflection on the prescribing skills of the practitioner.

Another assumption that can impede diagnosis and referral for treatment is the belief that older adults are not responsive to addiction treatment. By inference, we may draw a reasonable conclusion about treatment of older persons with drug abuse and dependence. It has been demonstrated that older adult alcoholics are more likely than the nonelderly to complete treatment and to have outcomes that are as good or better than younger patients (Atkinson, 1995). Until we have more data concerning treatment outcomes, the authors propose that we assume that much of the experience with alcoholism treatment can be translated to prescription drugs.

Case Studies Illustrating Treatment Strategies

The authors now present five clinical vignettes that illustrate different levels of care as conceptualized by the American Society of Addiction Medicine (ASAM) Patient Placement Criteria (1996). These criteria apply to treatment for psychoactive drug-related disorders and serve as a clinical guide to be used in matching patients to appropriate levels of care. There are other features of the criteria, but this chapter is too brief to consider them in detail. The ASAM manual also discusses dimensions other than level of service, the assessment process, the goals of intervention and treatment, informed consent, and other important aspects of using the criteria.

ASAM Levels of Service

Levels of service in the Patient Placement Criteria range from early intervention through outpatient services to medically managed intensive inpatient care (ASAM, 1996, page 5). Each level of care or service describes a range of resources available to be applied within a given period of time to addiction and related problems. The levels of service described in the Criteria are:

Level 0.5: Early Intervention
Level I: Outpatient Services
Level II: Intensive Outpatient/Partial Hospitalization Services
Level III: Residential/Inpatient Services
Level IV: Medically Managed Intensive Inpatient Services

Special attention will be given to the setting, range of services available, dimensions of service, and the continuing service and discharge criteria, whenever appropriate.

Case 1: ASAM Level 0.5 Early Intervention. A 69-year-old woman had recently lost her husband and requested a sleeping aid from her family physician. Lorazepam at bedtime for 2 weeks was prescribed. When the supply of lorazepam was exhausted and she was still having insomnia, she called the doctor and the prescription was renewed for another 2 weeks. The physician did not hear from her until she came in for an appointment 2 months later. She explained that she was still having insomnia when the second prescription of Lorazepam® had run out. She said that she didn't want to "bother you again." She recalled that her husband had been using Valium (diazepam, 5 mg) for sleep and upon searching his medication supply, she found a bottle of diazepam, numbering about 90 tablets. She began to use one at bedtime. Although her sleep improved, it became necessary to gradually increase the dose, up to 20 mg. daily. With this treatment of insomnia she became increasingly sleepless and "depressed." Other symptoms included anorexia with weight loss, fatigue, loss of interest, and social withdrawal. Suicidal ideation was absent.

The physician knew the patient well, including the fact that she had no prior history of depression and that her general physical condition had been good. Some routine laboratory studies were ordered, however, including thyroid function and a blood chemistry group. These results were normal or negative. She diagnosed the patient as having a major depression and set up a program for tapering off the diazepam. In addition the physician referred her to a grief support group. An antidepressant was started and she was counseled in the proper use of medications. She experienced an uneventful recovery over the course of about 3 months.

Comment: Although the patient had misused the benzodiazepine diazepam, there had not been a pattern of such behavior in the past and there was nothing else to suggest addictive traits. Major depression does occur quite commonly in the course of bereavement. To what extent benzodiazepines may have complicated the mood problem is open to conjecture, but it has been reported to occur. A primary care, office-based intervention was appropriate in this case. The physician and her office staff were sufficient for managing the problem and providing continuing care.

Case 2: ASAM Level I Outpatient Services. A physician was called by a local hospital emergency room physician and informed that one of his patients, a 78-year-old retired banker, had been brought in by ambulance. He had fallen and was injured while shopping in a nearby mall. The physician went to the ER and evaluated his patient. He had not been seriously injured, having "just a bad bruise" on his elbow. There were other contusions, however, of various ages. The patient admitted that he had been "more unsteady than usual for about a year." The physician suspected that his patient's use of diazepam (15 mg. daily) could have been the problem. The patient was advised to reduce the dose to 10 mg. daily, but not to stop it. Arrangements were made for a more complete exam to be done at the doctor's office the following week.

The physical and laboratory examination of the patient did not pinpoint a cause for the gait problem. This brought the discussion back to medication use. Diazepam had been started 25 years earlier when his wife threatened to leave him. What the patient had *not* told the physician was that she had threatened to leave him then. His efforts to reduce diazepam in the past had failed. Each time the patient complained that he couldn't sleep and "got the jitters" if the diazepam dose was reduced. The physician insisted that the patient be evaluated at a local outpatient addiction program. The patient reluctantly agreed after the doctor stated that he could not continue to care for him if he wouldn't accept his recommendations.

The independent evaluation confirmed a past history of alcohol dependence and current dependence on a benzodiazepine. A treatment plan was developed. The patient would gradually taper off the diazepam over the next 6 weeks. Periodic serum levels would be obtained to monitor compliance. He would also participate in twice weekly psychotherapy sessions in an addictions rehabilitation program over the next 8 weeks and his wife would also participate in a family program. The outpatient detoxification went smoothly except for one episode of "cheating" (with a benzodiazepine) by the patient. The psychotherapy helped the patient to accept the fact of his alcoholism and although he had stopped drinking, he had simply substituted one chemical dependence for another. He agreed to participate in Alcoholics Anonymous on a regular basis. The wife stated that she had benefited greatly and said, "I have my husband back." She agreed to attend Al Anon. The physician continued to see his patient at regular intervals and the addiction counselor did so as well for the first year of continuing care.

Comment: The chronic use of psychoactive drugs by persons known or suspected of having alcoholism (active or inactive) is cause for concern. Prior alcoholism is a risk factor for subsequent problematic dependence on benzodiazepines. In this case the past history of alcoholism was not previously revealed to the physician. The physician was correct in using pressure to obtain the patient's agreement to be evaluated at the addiction center. He recognized that there had been a relapse problem (brief unsuccessful attempts at reducing or stopping medication) and correctly identified the problem of resistance to treatment. The physician also recognized the need to utilize outside services to help his patient. The outpatient treatment staff drew upon community services, including AA and Al Anon to help the patient and his wife.

Case 3: ASAM Level II Intensive Outpatient/Partial Hospitalization Services. A married 61-year-old mother of four children, living with her spouse, had been having migraine headaches for as long as she could remember. When she was young her mother had brought her to the family doctor on many occasions seeking help for her. Numerous medications were tried, including barbiturates, opiates, and various hypnotics. The results were variable. When the patient married she started taking birth control pills and the episodic headaches improved. She remained stable for many years, even after stopping the birth control medication, with the use of small doses of opiates and various nonopioid analgesics. In her late 50s however, her only daughter was killed in an auto accident. She struggled with depressed moods and didn't accept a recommendation for psychotherapy because "that wouldn't bring my daughter back." Her use of the opiate codeine increased and tolerance developed as evidenced by increasingly higher doses needed to control the headaches. She became very protective of her supply. In addition, she had not followed the recommended dosing and had escalated the dose to about 250 mg. of codeine phosphate daily. On one occasion she explained that she had run out of medication early because she inadvertently "dropped the medication into the toilet" and on another occasion she said that she "lost it out in the snow."

A thorough general medical and neurological examination including head imaging yielded normal results. Psychiatric consultation led to a recommendation for admission to an outpatient addiction service. The patient, "desperate to try anything," accepted. Additional evaluation led to these DSM-IV-based diagnoses: Axis I: codeine dependence and psychogenic pain disorder, Axis III: migraine headaches. She was placed on a 3-week tapering schedule of codeine that was accomplished without any evidence of a withdrawal syndrome. Drug-seeking behavior was managed through support and psychotherapy. The latter focused on two broad issues, her persistent underlying anger about her daughter's death, and her denial concerning the dependence on an opiate. She revealed that she had not been truthful about the "lost" medication. In addition she began to understand the link between her head pain and the inner emotional "pain" which was related to her bereavement. She displayed considerable pain behavior during the group sessions, e.g., bending forward with her head in her hands, grimacing, moaning, and shifting positions. Parallel sessions were scheduled for her at a pain management unit nearby and her husband was included in the pain management counseling as he had been in the addiction sessions. He discovered that he had unwittingly been reinforcing his wife's perception that she needed more and more pain killer as well as responding to and maintaining her pain behavior. Continuing outpatient management was provided by the outpatient addiction program physician and counselor and community support groups. This included medical management of the patient's migraine headaches with non-addicting medication. The headaches returned to a typical episodic, migraine-like pattern, but were much less problematic.

Comment: Chronic pain frequently leads to prescription drug dependence, one of medicine's great conundrums. Physicians are sometimes tempted to simply supply the patient with all the medication that he or she demands. Attempting to handle such a problem in the practitioner's office setting can be a thoroughly frustrating experience and of little benefit to the patient. When an outpatient setting is deemed appropriate, as in the case described, the drug taper can be conducted over a longer time interval than would be required in an inpatient setting in which the primary goal for the taper is the avoidance of physiological withdrawal symptoms. A slow taper often helps the patient make the adjustment to a drug-free state more smoothly by minimizing psychological as well as physical distress. The length of the withdrawal should be individualized. The issue of resistance to treatment was partially resolved in this case even before admission by this patient who was "desperate to try anything." In summary the dimensions addressed during treatment had included: managing detoxification, providing non-drug alternatives for pain management, integrating medical treatment for migraine headaches into the addiction rehabilitation, providing psychotherapy for grief issues, and providing adequate medical treatment and counseling follow-up care.

Case 4: ASAM Level III Residential/Inpatient Service. An 82-year-old married Caucasian female was admitted on a voluntary basis to an inpatient addiction program for a first addiction treatment. Flurazepam (Dalmane®), a benzodiazepine, had been prescribed 7 years earlier for treatment of insomnia. Several months before admission she read a book which listed Dalmane as an addicting drug. She received contradictory advice from physicians concerning the drug, i.e., as to its ability to produce dependence. Eventually she stopped the drug and experienced increased anxiety, rapid heartbeat, excessive perspiration and tremors. She restarted the drug. Weeks later she was referred to a psychiatrist and attempts were made to withdraw the flurazepam on an outpatient basis, but without success. Except for persistent initial insomnia she denied core symptoms of major depression at the time of admission to the treatment center. She did have upper gastrointestinal symptoms, however.

The patient denied having misused the drug and did not describe other behaviors that were addictive in nature. She had also used butalbital (Fiorinal®), a barbiturate sedative, on a regular basis for many years for headaches but denied abuse. She had not used alcohol or nicotine. There was a past history of recurrent episodes of major depression requiring hospitalization on three occasions, the last being 7 years previously, the time when the flurazepam was started. There was no evidence of mental disorders in the family.

The mental status examination revealed a well-dressed and groomed woman who was talkative and actively engaging in reminiscence. Her affect was bright and her mood was normal. Her intelligence was estimated as average. A Folstein Mini-Mental-State-Exam revealed only minor disorientation to the day of the week. The physical examination was normal except for a slight heart murmur, well-healed abdominal surgical scars, and spinal scoliosis. A urine screen was positive for benzodiazepines. The Millon Clinical Multiaxial Inventory-II, a measure of personality traits, revealed a pattern of avoiding self-disclosure, with prominent elevation on the dependent and compulsive personality scales. Consultations and testing led to the clinical impression that the patient had dyspepsia and postprandial pain, secondary to gastroesophogeal reflux disorder (GERD) which she had had in the past. Adjustments in her gastrointestinal medications were recommended.

The multidisciplinary team summary generated the following problem list: (1) Risk of withdrawal syndrome from a long-acting benzodiazepine. (2) Patient had been unable to abstain from flurazepam. (3) Persisting symptoms of gastroesophogeal reflux disorder while on treatment.

The flurazepam was stopped to allow for a gradual elimination of the drug from the body under controlled conditions. This was possible because of the naturally slow elimination of this medication, especially in elderly persons. An abstinence syndrome (withdrawal) was not observed during a 14-day hospitalization. Trazodone was used to treat insomnia. The therapy focused on pain management, the doctor-patient relationship, reducing marital stress and building a network of support for abstinence from addicting drugs. Although she had insomnia, a diagnosis of major depression was not made during her hospital stay. G.I. medications were adjusted with good results. Headache improved. Her mood was normal and sleep was improved. The following discharge diagnoses (DSM-IV) were entered:

Axis I: benzodiazepine dependence, with physiological dependence,

Axis III: tension headaches, hypertension, aortic regurgitation, coronary artery disease, esophagitis secondary to gastroesophageal reflux disorder and degenerative joint disease,

Axis IV: medical illness and marital stress.

Continuing care arrangements required that the patient visit her internist in 5 days. An appointment was also made with an addiction psychiatrist, who, however, was not available for 2 months. She was instructed to continue trazodone 100 mg. daily at bedtime. She called the hospital treatment center 2 weeks after discharge to report that she had begun to experience insomnia, excessive sweating, rapid heartbeat, loss of appetite, and increased anxiety 1 week after the initial visit with her internist, at which time she had been stable. The senior physician and her internist conferred by telephone and she was seen by the internist that day. She was diagnosed as having late-onset benzodiazepine withdrawal and was treated with a clonidine 0.1mg patch that was successful in ameliorating the withdrawal syndrome. Five days later the insomnia problem had worsened and her internist increased the trazadone dose to 150 mg. She improved. At 79 days following hospital discharge she had not kept the appointment with the psychiatrist and was experiencing multiple physical symptoms and a dysphoric and anxious mood. An appointment with the psychiatrist was obtained and the examination led to a diagnosis of major depression. She was treated with sertraline (Zoloft®) 50 mg. daily. One year following hospital discharge she was well, taking sertraline 25 mg. and trazodone 50 mg. daily. She had not returned to the use of benzodiazepines.

Comment: We have included this case to illustrate two important aspects of the general problem of prescription drug dependence. The first of these is the problem of comorbidity, especially involving mental disorders. This older woman had been treated for major depression three times in the past and because of this history of recurrent depression she was a definite candidate for long-term antidepressant therapy, not to be confused with long-term sedative treatment that was given 7 years earlier in this case. Her clinical course presented challenges for the physicians involved well after the patient had completed her inpatient addiction treatment. Ongoing case management is needed in such cases just as it is with any other chronic medical disorder. It is a mistake to use "aftercare" thinking in the area of psychoactive prescription drug dependencies because it suggests that the treatment was completed.

Case 5: ASAM Level IV Medically Managed Intensive Inpatient Services. A 66-year-married man with a longstanding history of "panic disorder" was transferred to an inpatient addiction unit from a medical psychiatry unit for completion of drug detoxification and rehabilitation from an addictive disorder. At age 20, he had developed an anxiety disorder while at sea in the U.S. Navy. The disorder had elements of post-traumatic stress disorder and panic attacks. He had a choking episode while eating, after which he had panic attacks that he described as a sense of choking and breathing too fast. He received a service-connected disability for mental health reasons. He had been treated in VA hospitals and had been prescribed many benzodiazepines over the years.

The patient also had a history of chronic low-back pain starting at age 29. He suffered an accidental fall when he was 42, after which his pain worsened. He underwent two spinal surgeries in his late 40s, both of which offered only temporary relief. He had been using opiate (naturally occurring) and opioid (synthetic) narcotic analgesics intermittently since the onset of his back pain. By age 64 a morphine pump had been started. After exhausting all other possibilities, his physician implanted an intrathecal pump and changed to hydromorphone a few months before admission, following development of an allergy to morphine. At about that time the patient's wife noticed that he had mental changes, such as difficulties with memory and confusion, including disorientation. At the time he presented to the Mayo Clinic for evaluation, the patient was on the following medications:

Intrathecal hydromorphone, 8 mg per day for pain
Hydrocodone/acetaminophen, 5/500, 6 tablets daily for pain
Fluoxetine, 60 mg daily for depression
Nefazodone, 200 mg nightly for anxiety/depression
Doxepin, 50 mg nightly for insomnia
Clonazepam, 1 mg three times daily for anxiety
Methylphenidate, 60–90 mg daily for somnolence

The patient also had a past history of stroke at age 63, followed by episodes of confusion and slurred speech, which were thought to be transient ischemic attacks. He also had a history of elevated blood lipids and myocardial infarction, as well as duodenal ulcers. In addition to the already mentioned medications, the patient was on a medication to block stomach acid, a medication for high blood pressure, a blood lipid lowering agent, and entericcoated aspirin.

The evidence for opioid dependence included chronic, daily use with adverse effects, the development of tolerance, withdrawal syndrome, and drug-seeking behavior. Denial was an additional feature of his dependence. He said that he had abstained from alcohol following his first anxiety attack at age 20. Before that, he only drank one beer at a sitting on an occasional basis. He was a smoker with a 45-pack-year history. He drank approximately 3–4 cups of caffeinated coffee daily. The family psychiatric history was significant for a brother who had schizophrenia and had committed suicide.

At the time of evaluation the patient could identify himself, but not others, nor could he correctly identify the place and date. He demonstrated lability of mood and affect, being alternatively irritable, sad, and tearful. Speech and language mechanisms were intact. Thought form was tangential, and content focused on his continuing pain symptoms and fear of discontinuing any of his analgesics or anxiolytics. The history was positive for intermittent suicidal ideation, but he had no particular plan in mind. He was an inpatient on the medical psychiatry unit for 2 weeks, during which time the intrathecal hydromorphone was reduced by 1 mg per day, every 3 days. The fluoxetine, nefazedone, and doxepin were tapered and discontinued, and the methylphenidate was stopped. The clonazepam was tapered to a total of 2 mg daily in three divided doses. The patient tolerated the initial part of his detoxification very well. It became evident that he had been suffering from a drug-induced, intoxication delirium (confusion). During this phase of treatment, he became more mentally clear and his ability to speak and think in an organized fashion improved dramatically. His mood was no longer depressed, and he denied suicidal thoughts. He did, however, struggle against the plan to continue tapering the antianxiety and pain medication. He complained that his pain continued unabated, although it did not worsen as the analgesics were tapered. He also expressed resentment that people considered him "addicted" to the medications, stating that he only took what his doctor had prescribed, and never deviated from directions for administration. He reluctantly agreed to inpatient addiction treatment to complete the taper of his medications and participate in the rehabilitation program. The patient and his wife had a great deal of difficulty accepting that he was drug dependent. The drug withdrawals were completed successfully and strategies were developed to help him manage his anxiety and chronic pain without resorting to the use of addicting substances.

Comment: This patient's case illustrates several factors that put the elderly at risk for drug abuse. These were: (1) The presence of a mental disorder, in this case an anxiety disorder. (2) History of daily use of multiple psychoactive drugs. (3) An injury followed by a chronic pain disorder. His misuse of prescription drugs was only identified after he had been experiencing slurred speech, mental status changes, and confusion. Sometimes these problems are attributed to "normal" aging or a medical condition. The symptoms of slurred speech and mental status changes including confusion were originally attributed to transient ischemic attacks, in the context of his history of cerebrovascular disease and stroke.

The patient had seen several physicians who were treating him and gave him access to his medications: a primary care physician, a psychiatrist, and a pain specialist. Having a primary care physician as well as one or more specialists is not an uncommon scenario for older adults, who have an increased incidence and prevalence of major chronic medical disorders associated with advancing age.

The chronic pain condition grew worse as this man aged, contributing to heightened anxiety. He thought that he had no other alternative than to take more medications to relieve his symptoms. This case underscores the importance of obtaining a complete medication list and updating it at each office visit. If the patient is vague about medication names and doses, the physician should request that the patient bring in all of the medication bottles to each office visit so they can be carefully reviewed.

Lastly, the withdrawal methods employed for several classes of prescription medications varied. Hydromorphone was tapered using its current route of administration, an intrathecal catheter and pump. The stimulant methylphenidate was stopped. SSRI antidepressants were tapered to reduce the risk of a serotonin withdrawal reaction. Clonazepam was tapered using oral dosing. Some of the withdrawals carried over into the inpatient addiction treatment portion of the patient's hospitalization. The topic of detoxification cannot be addressed in detail in this chapter; however, the authors have provided Tables 9.1 and 9.2 as a resource to aid in planning for withdrawal of the most common of the dependency producing drugs, benzodiazepines, opiates, and opioids.

Table 9.1 Benzodiazepines and Phenobarbital Substitution Dose Equivalents for Managing Withdrawal

Generic Name	Trade Name	Therapeutic Dose Range (mg/day)[a]	Half-life in hours	Equivalent dose to 30 mg phenobarbital
alprazolam	Xanax	0.5–4	12±2	
chlordiazepoxide	Librium	15–100	10±3.4	25
clonazepam	Klonopin	0.5–4	23±5	1
clorazepate	Tranxene	15–60	2±0.9	30
diazepam	Valium	5–40	43±13	10
flurazepam	Dalmane	15–30	15±5	30
lorazepam	Ativan	1–6	14±5	2
oxazepam	Serax	30–90	8±2.4	30
quazepam	Doral	7.5–15	39	15
temazepam	Restoril	7.5–30	11±6	15
triazolam	Halcion	0.125–0.50	2.9±1.0	0.1+25

Note. From Baldessarini (1996); Benet & Schwartz (1996); Hobbs, Rall, & Verdoon (1996); Schatzberg, Cole, & DeBattista (1997); Smith & Wesson, (1999). Adapted with permission.

[a]Dosing should be adjusted based upon the patient's age and medical condition.

Table 9.2 Opiate/Opioid Equivalent Doses for Managing Withdrawal

Generic Name	Trade Name	Dose in Mg.[a]	Half-life (in hours)
codeine		200	2–3
heroin		5 IM	0.5
hydromorphone	Dilaudid	7.5	2–3
hydrocodone	Lortab and Vicodin (with acetaminophen)	5–10[b]	2–4
methadone	Dolophine	10 IM 20 p.o	12–>150
morphine		20–60	2–3
morphine, controlled release	MS Contin Oramorph SR	20–60	2–3
oxycodone	Percodan	20–30	2–3
propoxyphene	Darvon	65	6–12

Note. From Portenoy & Payne (1997); and Reisne & Pasternak (1996). Adapted with permission.

[a]Doses are oral unless otherwise specified. The doses listed are equianalgesic doses to a parenteral dose of 10 mg of morphine. These ratios are useful when switching drugs; when switching, reduce the dose of the newly introduced drug by 25–50% to account for incomplete cross-tolerance.

[b]The equianalgesic dose of the compound refers to the opioid component only.

Some Additional Thoughts About Treatment Models

We find that the medical literature has largely focused on psychoactive prescription drug misuse within the context of side effects and complications. Very little research has addressed prescription drug use by the elderly within the framework of addictive disorders. Elderly persons seldom present to mental health clinics or hospitals for help with such disorders. They are much more likely to see their family doctor, internist, or other physicians who provide their general care. Of those who are diagnosed as having a drug abuse or addictive disorder, it is likely that few are referred for formal treatment. The study by Finlayson and Davis (1994) examined the records of over seven thousand adult patients who had been admitted to the Mayo Clinic's inpatient addiction treatment unit over a period of 20 years. Of these 11% were elderly and 16% of these had been dependent on a psychoactive prescription drug, some in combination with alcohol. Data collection was stopped with 100 elderly persons who had been diagnosed as having prescription drug dependence only. Psychiatric disorders were common in the study group. The most common were mood disorders (32%), organic mental disorders

(28%), personality disorders (27%), somatoform disorders (16%), and anxiety disorders (12%). If our experience with inpatients is representative of the general elderly population at risk, psychiatric disorders may be the main pathway to drug dependence in the elderly.

Age and the drug culture are important considerations in choosing a treatment setting. The assumption that the elderly addict might be best treated in a group of his/her peers is rational. Clinical experience teaches us that many elderly have difficulty relating to young addicts, especially those who use street drugs and have problems with the law. They come from different drug cultures. This culture may in fact be more important than the age factor. The street drug abuser is typically young and uses drugs to "get high" or to stave off withdrawal, and is involved in illegal activity, in some cases dealing in drugs. The medical profession is largely outside the sphere of their activities. The older adult prescription drug user, with the exception of users of diverted prescription drugs, is involved with medical practitioners and pharmacists, is operating within the law, and does not seek drugs to "get high." These are major factors, bound to affect perceptions of use, psychological defenses, and motivation to stop abuse, etc. Drug use could be as important or more important than age *per se*. This is a potentially fruitful area for future research.

There is another helpful concept of treatment and management that is germane to the idea of drug addiction. The prescription drug-dependent person with psychiatric and other medical issues usually has ongoing contact with physicians, nurses, and others operating within the medical realm. Insomnia, chronic pain, falls with injuries, anxiety, and depressed moods will be the main reasons for recontact with health professionals. These will be the multiple clinical problems and professional contacts occurring over time, referred to by some as the patient's *clinical pathway* (Kitchiner et al., 1996). Finlayson (1998) has discussed the potential benefit of using case management and paying attention to clinical pathways for care of the elderly drug-dependent person. In its most simple form the concept of clinical pathways (sometimes referred to as "critical pathways") posits that, as with most illnesses, drug dependence follows a course in which adverse events can be anticipated and their management planned. The allocation of resources is more or less spread uniformly over the course of the illness, rather than focusing on a specific period as "the treatment" or by the patient as "my treatment."

We have, up to this point, emphasized the importance of the prescription drug culture and the clinical pathway as useful concepts in the management of the older prescription drug-dependent person. Research reported to date does not, however, establish the best model for addressing the *core features* of this addiction. We refer to denial, somatization, chronic pain behavior, depression, and enabling behavior by others, etc. It has been the authors' experience that most elderly persons with prescription drug dependence are treated initially in mainline adult programs. Many of these utilize the Alcoholics Anonymous "12-step" model for alcohol as well as other drugs. Judging by the relatively small number of elderly with prescription drug problems who are admitted to addiction programs and the lack of published research in the area, we might assume that most of the experience in treatment of these elderly has been on this basis. The relative efficacy of 12-step programs in treating alcoholism was affirmed by the Project MATCH Research Group (1997). Twelve-step philosophy and programs are closely identified with the "Minnesota Model," involving 28 days of treatment in either a hospital or residential-based program. Following the treatment, the patient enters "aftercare." This implies that "treatment" has been administered, after which the patient will have "care." The risk involved in this thinking is that less emphasis may be placed on the "aftercare" than is actually needed. A rigid adherence to this thinking runs contrary to what we have been emphasizing up to this point.

A closer examination of the Minnesota Model and 12–step thinking reveals that, at its core, it is not inconsistent with clinical pathways thinking. J. Spicer, President of Hazeldon Foundation (1993) stated in his book, *The Minnesota Model: The Evolution of the Multidisciplinary Approach to Addiction Recovery.* "We need assessments that plot the individual's experience of sobriety on a continuum...." What we authors are attempting to accomplish by bringing in the concepts of drug culture, clinical pathways, and the 12 steps is to suggest a framework for treating the elderly prescription drug-dependent person utilizing familiar resources widely available to the typical clinician. The result is efficient use of hospital stays, ongoing case management by primary care physicians or professional case managers, forward-looking treatment planning, psychiatric care as indicated, addiction counseling, peer group support, and the application of 12-step concepts.

The practice, once common, of admitting persons with addictive disorders to residential or hospital-based programs has yielded to managed-care pressures and research-based evidence that outpatient treatment is effective for some levels of severity of the illness. Hospital stays for primary treatment of addiction are now largely reserved for detoxification, stabilization of various medical disorders, management of suicidality, and other acute problems. Partial hospitalization and outpatient programs are increasingly being used for most rehabilitation efforts with addicts. This reduces cost or allows available financial resources to be spread over a longer time period. This is consistent with the medical model of addiction, i.e., it is a chronic, relapsing disorder, for which a cure is not known, but can brought into remission at the time of diagnosis or at times of relapse. This understanding is compatible with the case management and clinical pathway paradigms. To use a comparison from general medicine, not all patients with diabetes mellitus require hospitalization at the time of diagnosis and some are never hospitalized. When hospitalization does occur it is for a specific purpose, enabling the patient to return to outpatient, long-term management. Critical events, nodal points as it were, occur and require an adjustment in intensity of care. With such a model financial and human resources can be used in an efficient manner.

Summary

1. Elderly persons are at risk for prescription drug dependence as a result of medical and psychiatric comorbidity.
2. Care often comes from multiple providers, thereby adding complexity to prescribing patterns and supervision.
3. Denial and shame may interfere with the patient and his/her family's motivation and resolve to follow a treatment plan.
4. Relapse to benzodiazepine and opioid use is common.
5. The complexity and risk of relapse are best addressed by having someone take charge of the case, i.e., a particular physician or another case manager who is prepared to identify critical nodal points along the clinical pathway and respond to them based upon a plan which has anticipated adverse outcomes.
6. "Aftercare" thinking should give way to a medical model in which the need for ongoing, *active care* is provided for these complex patients.

References

American Psychiatric Association. (1994). *Diagnostic and statistical manual of mental disorders* (4th ed.). Washington, DC: Author.

American Society of Addiction Medicine, Inc. (1996). *Patient placement criteria for the treatment of substance-related disorders,* (2nd ed.), Chevy Chase, MD: American Society of Addiction Medicine, Inc.

Atkinson, R. (1995). Treatment programs for aging alcoholics. In T. Beresford, & E. Gomberg (Editors), *Alcohol and aging,* (pp. 186–210). New York: Oxford University Press.

Baldessasrini, R. (1996). Drugs in the treatment of psychiatric disorders. In J. G. Hardman, L. L. Limbird, P. B. Molinoff, R. W. Ruddon, & A. G. Gillman (Editors), *Goodman & Gilman's, the pharmacological basis of therapeutics* (9th ed.). New York: McGraw-Hill.

Benet, L. Z., Oie, S., & Schwartz, J. B. (1996). Design and optimization of dosage regimens; pharmacokinetic data. In J. G. Hardman, L. L. Limbird, P. B. Molinoff, R. W. Ruddon, & A. G. Gillman (Editors), *Goodman and Gilman's, the pharmacological basis of therapeutics* (9th ed.). New York: McGraw-Hill.

Finlayson, R. E. (1997). Misuse of prescription drugs. In A. G. Gurnack (Editor), *Older adults' misuse of alcohol, medicines, and other drugs* (pp. 158–184). New York: Springer Publishing.

Finlayson, R. E. (1998). Prescription drug dependence in the elderly: The clinical pathway to recovery. *Journal of Mental Health and Aging, 4,* 233–249.

Finlayson, R. E., & Davis, L. J. (1994). Prescription drug dependence in the elderly population: Demographic and clinical features of 100 inpatients. *Mayo Clinic Proceedings, 69,* 1137–1145.

Hasday, J. D., & Karch, F. E. (1981). Benzodiazepine prescribing in a family medicine center. *Journal of the American Medical Association, 256,* 1321–1325.

Hobbs, W. R., Rall, T. W., & Verdoon, T. A. (1996). Hypnotics and sedatives; alcohol. In J. G. Hardman, L. L. Limbird, P. B. Molinoff, R. W. Ruddon, & A. G. Gillman (Editors), *Goodman & Gilman's, the pharmacological basis of therapeutics* (9th ed.). New York: McGraw-Hill.

Holroyd, S., & Duryee, J. J. (1997). Substance use disorders in a geriatric psychiatry outpatient clinic: Prevalence and epidemiologic characteristics. *Journal of Nervous & Mental Disease, 185*(10), 627–632.

Kitchiner, D., Davidson, C., & Dundred, P. (1996). Integrated care pathways: Effective tools for continuous evaluation of clinical practice. *Journal of Evaluation in Clinical Practice, 2*(1), 65–69.

North, D. A., McAvoy, B. R., & Powell, A. M. (1992). Benzodiazepine use in general practice: Is it a problem? *New Zealand Medical Journal, 105,* 287–289.

Portenoy, R. K., & Payne, R. (1997). Acute and chronic pain, In J. H. Lowinson, P. Ruiz, R. B. Millman, & J. G. Langrod (Editors), *Substance abuse: A comprehensive textbook.* Baltimore: Williams and Wilkins.

Project MATCH Research Group. (1997). Matching alcoholism treatment to client heterogeneity: Project MATCH posttreatment drinking outcomes. *Journal of Studies in Alcoholism 58*(1), 7–20.

Reisne, T., & Pasternak, G. (1996). Opioid analgesics and antagonists. In J. G. Hardman, L. L. Limbird, P. B. Molinoff, R. W. Ruddon, & A. G. Gillman (Editors), *Goodman & Gilman's, the pharmacological basis of therapeutics* (9th ed.). New York: McGraw-Hill.

Ried, L. D., Johnson, R. E., & Gettman, D. A. (1998). Benzodiazepine exposure and functional status in older people. *The Journal of the American Geriatrics Society, 46,* 71–76.

Schatzberg, A. F., Cole, J. O., & DeBattista, C. (1997). *Manual of Clinical Pharmacology.* Washington, DC: American Psychiatric Press.

Shorr, R. I., Bauwens, S. F., & Landefeld, C. S. (1990). Failure to limit quantities of benzodiazepine hypnotic drugs for outpatients: Placing the elderly at risk. *American Journal of Medicine, 89,* 725–732.

Smith, D. E., & Wesson, D. R. (1999). Benzodiazepines and other sedative-hypnotics. In M. Galanter, & H. Kleber (Editors), *Textbook of substance abuse treatment* (2nd ed.). Washington, DC: American Psychiatric Press.

Spicer, J. (1993). *The Minnesota Model: The evolution of the the multidisciplinary approach to addiction recovery.* Center City, MN: Hazeldon Foundation.

Wesson, D. R., & Smith, D. E. (1990). Prescription drug abuse: Patient, physician, and cultural responsibilities. *Western Journal of Medicine, 152,* 613–616.

10

Smoking Cessation for Older Smokers

Neal R. Boyd and C. Tracy Orleans

Introduction

Many smoking cessation programs have been developed and targeted to various segments of the smoking population since the first *Surgeon General's Report on Smoking and Health* in 1964 (USDHEW, 1964). Only recently, however, has attention been directed to the needs of midlife and older smokers, defined in this chapter as those age 50 years and older. Smokers in this age group began smoking when smoking was considered a glamorous part of the American social culture and long before its health consequences were well known. The result is a generation of lifelong heavy smokers. With more baby boomers reaching midlife, the ranks of older smokers are on the rise (Orleans, 1997). Older smokers not only experience significant health consequences from continued smoking but derive many important health benefits from quitting. However, after several decades of smoking, older smokers who attempt quitting encounter barriers somewhat different from those faced by smokers in younger age groups. This chapter reviews the smoking problem among midlife and older smokers and offers strategies for successfully intervening with this population.

Table 10.1 Smoking and the Leading Causes of Death for Age 65 and Older[a]

Heart Disease
Cancer
Cerebrovascular Disease
Chronic Obstructive Pulmonary Disease
Pneumonia and Influenza
Diabetes Mellitus
Accidents
Alzheimer's Disease
Nephritis
Septicemia

[a]Diseases for which smoking is a risk factor are **bolded**.

Health Consequences of Smoking

Currently, more than 13 million people over age 50 smoke (Shopland et al., 1996). The smoking prevalence rate among those over age 50 constitutes about 27% of the U.S. smoking population (CDC, 1996). Annually, over 400,000 Americans die from cigarette smoking, with approximately 94% of these smoking-related deaths occurring after age 50 (CDC, 1996). In fact, as shown in Table 10.1, smoking is a risk factor in 6 of the top 10 causes of death for those age 65 years and older (Ventura & Smith, 1998). Smoking significantly increases the likelihood of morbidity and mortality from numerous diseases, including cardiovascular and cerebrovascular, respiratory diseases, and cancers of the lung, larynx, pharynx, bladder, kidney, pancreas, and cervix (Shopland & Burns, 1993). It also complicates many illnesses and conditions common among older people, including heart disease, high blood pressure, circulatory and vascular conditions, duodenal ulcers, osteoporosis, periodontal disease, age-related macular degeneration, cataracts, lens opacities, and diabetes (Boyd & Orleans, 1999). In addition, smoking interacts with and restricts the effectiveness of many medications that are used to treat many of these conditions (Moore, 1986).

Health Benefits of Quitting Smoking

Scientific evidence confirms (USDHHS, 1990) that quitting smoking leads to significant health benefits regardless of age. Thus, older adults who have smoked for decades reap substantial medical and psychological benefits from stopping smoking. Quitting smoking can prevent or reduce the likelihood of many diseases such as heart disease, cancer, and respiratory diseases (Shopland & Burns, 1993). Cessation can stabilize existing conditions such as chronic obstructive pulmonary disease. Giving up smoking in the later years can not only extend life, but also promotes a greater level of independent functioning (Fries, Green, & Levine 1989; Rimer & Orleans, 1993).

Beliefs About Smoking Among Older Smokers

In addition to a higher daily smoking rate compared with groups of younger smokers, older smokers have a different set of beliefs about smoking. An evaluation of the Adult Use of Tobacco Survey (AUTS) (Orleans, Jepson, Resch, & Rimer, 1994) compared smokers' beliefs about smoking in two age categories: the 21–49-year-old age group and the 50–74-year-old age group. Smokers age 50–74 years were not as likely as those age 21–49 years to believe that there is a relationship between smoking and illness. Moreover, the older group was not as concerned about the health consequences of smoking and was more skeptical about the benefits of smoking cessation. Older smokers were more likely to consider smoking as a means to cope with stress and control weight. Surprisingly, approximately one-half of these older smokers believed that smoking was not as much of a health risk as being 20 pounds overweight.

Not all of the evaluation of AUTS data was negative. The analysis did find a strong positive relationship between the beliefs about the health consequences of smoking and a physician's advice to quit (Orleans et al., 1994). Older smokers who reported having been advised by a doctor to quit were more likely to believe they were at risk for smoking-related diseases than those reporting not having received quitting advice from a clinician. Also, a positive relationship was found between older smokers' intentions to quit and physician advice to quit (Orleans et al., 1994). While these findings are only statistically significant relationships, they do suggest that clinician advice about smoking, health risks, and the offer of quitting strategies represents potentially powerful intervention strategies for older smokers. This is especially true given focus group findings that older smokers often underestimate not just the harms of smoking but the benefits of quitting (Rimer et al., 1994).

Rationale for Intervening With Older Smokers

At the time the United States Surgeon General (USDHHS, 1990) declared that "it is never too late to quit smoking," little was known about smoking cessation for older smokers (Orleans, 1997). During the past decade, the results of intervention research among older smokers has provided substantial evidence that older smokers are as likely, and possibly even more likely, than smokers in younger age groups to quit when given appropriate assistance (Orleans, 1997). The research showed that the predictors of quitting success for older smokers are similar to those identified for smokers in younger age groups. Factors found to be associated with quitting success include lower level nicotine dependence; higher quitting self-efficacy (see Fleming's and Dupree & Schonfeld's chapters); prior quitting success; stronger quitting motivation; greater perceived health benefits; lower perceived quitting barriers; using a greater number of quitting strategies; having few, if any, acquaintances who smoke and/or a nonsmoking spouse; and for older smokers using transdermal nicotine to quit, having more frequent contact with physicians, pharmacists, or both, and less smoking while wearing the patch (Orleans, 1997). Based on these data, it appears that older smokers are highly responsive to targeted smoking cessation programs.

The United States government has made considerable effort to reduce tobacco use in this country. The United States Department of Health and Human Services has included major tobacco control initiatives as a part of its Healthy People Objectives for the Nation for the years 1990, 2000, and 2001. The Year 2010 initiative continues the effort to reduce overall smoking prevalence in all age groups and to increase the proportion of physicians and other health professionals who routinely ask thc smoking status of all patients they see and counsel those who smoke to quit. In 1996 the Agency for Health Care Policy and Research (this organization is now known as the Agency for Health Care Research and Quality) issued clinical guidelines for smoking cessation. These guidelines, intended for physicians, smoking cessation specialists, health care administrators, insurers, and purchasers, were based on scientific evidence, and advocate routinely identifying and documenting tobacco users and delivery and support of effective tobacco cessation interventions in clinical practice.

Although specific recommendations for clinic-based smoking cessation exist, not all physicians intervene with their patients who smoke. A survey among older smokers revealed that only about one-half had ever been asked by their doctor about their smoking habits (USDHHS, 1990). Another survey of 50–74-year-old smokers revealed that nearly two-thirds were thinking about quitting in the next year (Rimer, Orleans, Keintz, et al., 1990). With older adults making an average of 6.3 physician visits a year, there are approximately 1.5 million annual physician encounters with older smokers who have never been advised to quit (Rimer & Orleans, 1990). If only 10% of these smokers could be motivated to quit by their health care provider, more than one million adults over age 50 would become ex-smokers annually (Rimer & Orleans, 1990).

Barriers to Intervention With Older Smokers

Many barriers exist to intervention with older adults who smoke. Compared with smokers in younger age groups, older smokers tend to be heavier smokers, smoking more than 20 cigarettes per day (Rimer & Orleans, 1993). This smoking rate leads to higher levels of nicotine addiction. Also, as we have already mentioned, older smokers are *less likely* than younger smokers to *believe in the health consequences of smoking* and less likely to believe that common smoking-related symptoms, such as shortness of breath or impaired functioning, are related to smoking (USDHHS, 1990). They are also more likely to report that smoking is a ritual that they have grown to enjoy and look forward to. To overcome barriers such as these is essential in successfully intervening with this group.

Efficacy of Physician-Initiated Interventions

Although health care practitioners have not routinely intervened to help their patients quit smoking, a number of randomized smoking cessation trials have been successfully conducted in physician offices for smokers of all ages. A review of 28 trials found that brief advice or counseling to stop smoking produced cessation rates of 5%–10% while more intensive interventions resulted in 20%–25% quit rates (Glynn, 1988). An analysis of National Cancer Institute (NCI)-funded smoking cessation trials involving over 30,000 patients and over 1,000 primary care providers revealed that smokers receiving physician-initiated interventions had long-term quit rates 2–6 times higher than patients receiving the usual care (Glynn & Manley, 1990). Although these studies involved smokers in all age groups, a recently completed physician office smoking cessation trial for smokers aged 50–74 years demonstrates that intervening with older smokers results in cessation outcomes comparable to those observed in other mixed-age, clinic-based smoking cessation evaluations (Morgan et al., 1996). This randomized trial compared usual care with a physician-delivered intervention. Thirty-nine outpatient medical practices recruited 659 older smokers to participate. Quit rates six months after the intervention were nearly twice as high for patients receiving the physician intervention than for patients in usual care: 15.4% versus 8.2%. By 12-months the physician intervention group abstinence rate had increased to 19.5% while the usual care group abstinence rate had increased to 12.9%.

Not only do physician-initiated interventions increase the likelihood of smoking cessation, but they are also cost-effective. Cummings and colleagues (1988) have estimated that provider advice to quit is as cost-effective as other preventive interventions, such as treating hypertension and hypercholesterolemia. Cost-benefit analyses are likely to be even greater in the presence of chronic disease. For example, Krumholz and colleagues (1993) estimated that smoking cessation is 20–200 times more cost-effective than standard medical therapies after acute myocardial infarction.

Components of Successful Intervention

The recently updated smoking cessation clinical guideline proposed a "5 As" model. The elements of this treatment strategy are:

1) *Ask* about and document smoking status (tobacco use) at every patient contact;
2) *Advise* all smokers (tobacco users) to quit;
3) *Assess* willingness to make a quit attempt;
4) *Assist* smokers' attempts to quit with self-help cessation materials and pharmacotherapy if indicated; and
5) *Arrange* for follow-up support to assess outcome and provide additional assistance if needed.

Effective smoking cessation interventions include several core components. These are: a 3–10 minute physician message to quit smoking, including setting a quit date; self-help materials presenting state of the art motivational, behavioral, and relapse prevention strategies; arranging for follow-up support; and prescriptions for pharmacotherapy, if indicated (Fiore, Bailey, Cohen, et al., 2000). (See a partial listing of self-help resources and where they may be obtained at the end of this chapter).

The Process of Quitting

It is important to understand that to quit smoking involves a process of behavioral change. Prochaska and DiClemente (1983) have developed a framework known as the Transtheoretical Model to understand how smokers quit. According to this model, smokers succeed at stopping smoking by advancing through a sequence of five motivational and behavioral change stages. These are: (1) precontemplation—not currently thinking about quitting smoking; (2) contemplation—seriously planning on quitting in the next 6 months; (3) preparation—planning to quit in the next month with at least one quit attempt in the previous year; (4) action—stopping smoking; and (5) maintenance—begins after having quit for 6 months and includes staying smoke free and resisting relapse. (This model has also been adapted for reducing alcohol consumption and is described in greater detail in chapter 6.) Often smokers find they must recycle through the stages in repeated efforts to quit smoking. Studies have found that different motivational and behavioral self-change processes are important in different stages of quitting (see chapter 6). More recently, intervention research has illustrated that stage-matched treatments produced greater quitting outcomes than stage mismatched treatments (Prochaska, DiClemente, Velicer, & Ross, 1993). Thus, it is very important to assess the smoker's stage of change as a part of the smoking history evaluation and apply an intervention suited to the stage of quitting readiness.

Pharmacologic Considerations

Nicotine replacement therapy is important for older smokers because most are highly addicted to nicotine. Nicotine polacrilex (gum) and transdermal nicotine patches are available over-the-counter without the need for a prescription from a health provider. When used appropriately nicotine gum helps alleviate many nicotine withdrawal symptoms that are commonly cited by older smokers (Orleans et al., 1994), including irritability, restlessness, anxiety, and difficulty concentrating (Fiore, Smith, Jorenby, & Baker, 1994; Silagy, Mant, Fowler, & Lodge, 1994). To be effective, nicotine gum must be chewed properly. Unlike regular chewing gum, nicotine gum should be chewed slowly and then "parked" between the cheek and gum to release nicotine. This possibly could be problematic for older smokers who wear dentures or have bridgework. However, Schneider (1987) has indicated that many older smokers can successfully use nicotine gum even in the presence of dentures or bridgework.

When nicotine gum is not chewed properly, it often causes unpleasant side effects such as a burning sensation in the throat, nausea, and gas. These side effects often lead to a lack of adherence to recommended regimens (Fiore et al., 1994; Silagy et al., 1994). Some studies (Silagy et al., 1994) have shown these effects were related to poor outcomes when used in the context of a brief medical advice intervention. Thus, when recommended within a brief physician context, doctors should allow time for adequate instruction in appropriate gum use.

Research on transdermal nicotine (Fiore et al., 1994) suggests the latter may be more effective in the context of routine physician interventions. This research suggests that the patch appears to benefit smokers at all levels of addiction. Appropriate use produces smoking cessation rates two to three times higher than those for brief medical advice alone. Ease of adherence and fewer side effects were two reasons attributed to superior efficacy of the patch. A survey (Orleans et al., 1994) of older patch users indicates that instruction in use is important for optimal benefit. Only about half of this study's patients reported that they had received any advice on patch use or quitting from their physician or pharmacist. This survey also revealed that the amount of provider instruction in use was significantly related to higher quit rates and lower rates of smoking while using the patch. Important use tips include wearing a new patch each day; not skipping a day; placing the patch at a different site on the body each day; and not smoking while wearing the patch.

In July 1996, the FDA approved nicotine gum and nicotine patches for over-the-counter (OTC) sales. While the OTC status of these medications will increase their availability, physicians and pharmacists must continue to intervene responsibly when recommending these aids. For one thing, these nicotine delivery methods may complicate the health status of patients who suffer from cardiovascular disease or diabetes mellitus, and may be contraindicated in some patients. And, as described above, doctors and pharmacists must deliver specific advice regarding proper utilization of these products. As OTC medication, nicotine replacement is expensive. Its high price may lead some potential users to conclude that either is not affordable. This is especially true for older smokers on limited income. When the cost issue arises, the cost-effectiveness of using nicotine replacement versus the expense of continuing smoking should be emphasized. A pack-a-day smoker quitting via nicotine replacement will more than pay for the medication with money saved from not having to purchase cigarettes during the next year. Also, the cost of using nicotine replacement is not nearly as expensive as the cost of more frequent physician visits for the various smoking-associated ailments throughout the coming years.

Recently bupropion hydrochloride, an antidepressant medication, marketed under the name of Zyban®, has been used effectively to help smokers quit. Research with bupropion as a pharmacologic treatment for smoking cessation is limited. Initial study suggests that it rivals the transdermal nicotine patch in effectiveness (Hurt et al., 1997). The attractiveness of this medication is that it does utilize nicotine for success. Bupropion works by triggering a brain response that is similar to that caused by nicotine. However, it is not addictive. At the present time it is unclear whether bupropion is an appropriate smoking cessation medication for older smokers. Research has documented that the elderly metabolize drugs at a slower rate than younger people. In addition, they are more sensitive to drug side effects (Lipman, 1985). Zyban is not recommended if the smoker is already taking another medication that is known to interact with bupropion. Given that older age groups consume the largest quantities of prescription medication, a careful review of an older individual's drug regimen is essential prior to prescribing Zyban for an older smoker.

Case Studies

Case 1. Tom S., age 71, was a new patient who had transferred from another medical group when his physician died. His initial visit was for a physical examination. He completed an extensive medical history and responded to a smoking history questionnaire. Of particular concern in Tom's medical history were hypertension and diabetes, both of which were controlled by prescription medication. He complained of shortness of breath when walking with his friends. Tom had been a smoker for 56 years and had smoked a pack and a half of cigarettes a day for most of his smoking life. He also smoked his first cigarette of the day within 30 minutes of awakening—a sign of high nicotine dependence. Tom expressed no interest in quitting smoking and did not believe in a relationship between smoking and illness. When advised that he should quit smoking, Tom was surprised. In a conversation about smoking, he explained that since he had smoked practically all his life, he believed that to stop smoking now would be giving up a pleasure that he had grown to look forward to. He said that he had heard the usual punitive reasons for quitting smoking many times and was actually skeptical. However, Tom acknowledged that he was unaware that the shortness of breath that he experienced when he walked with his friends was not due to aging as he had thought but to his smoking habit. Also, the information that smoking restricted the effectiveness of the medications he took to control hypertension and diabetes made him question whether he should continue smoking. The rewards that were described to Tom, such as being able to walk with friends without tiring quickly, and the possibility of not having to continue adjusting his prescription medication, he considered to be real benefits. A follow-up letter to Tom reinforced the benefits of quitting. As a result he returned to the office for assistance in planning a quit-smoking program. Tom preferred to quit with minimal assistance, as do most smokers. He was shown how to use *Clear Horizons,* a self-help smoking cessation guide designed for older smokers. This included use of prequitting strategies, such as setting a quit date, nicotine fading (i.e., switching to brands of cigarettes with progressively less nicotine), and social support. Given his nicotine dependence level, nicotine replacement therapy was strongly recommended, the cost of which was covered by his health insurance plan. Within one year Tom was an ex-smoker.

Comment: Assessment of Tom's initial stage of quitting readiness showed that he was a "precontemplator"—not interested in quitting—when he was first approached. The key to his quit attempt was relating his current health problems to his smoking habit and emphasizing the rewards that result from smoking cessation. Many older smokers need more discussion about the benefits of smoking cessation when assessing whether they are ready to try to quit. In fact, the updated clinical practice guideline (Fiore et al., 2000) recommends application of the "5 Rs" when smokers remain uninterested in quitting (see Table 10.2). In Tom's case, the additional discussion and follow-up reinforcement via letter led to a quit attempt that would not have happened otherwise.

Table 10.2 The 5 Rs to Enhance Motivation to Quit Smoking

Relevance	Make information relevant to the smoker's health condition, health concerns, family or social situation, age, and gender.
Risks	Ask the smoker to identify the health consequences and highlight those that are pertinent to the smoker.
Rewards	Ask the smoker to identify the benefits of quitting and highlight those that are particularly relevant to the smoker.
Roadblocks	Ask the smoker to identify the barriers that impede quitting and address each barrier.
Repetition	This type of motivational intervention should be repeated each time an unmotivated smoker makes an office visit.

Case 2. Alice P., age 67, had smoked more than a pack of cigarettes a day for 53 years. Alice's weight was well within a normal range as was her blood pressure. She had no history of chronic health problems and she considered herself to be very healthy. At the time of her office visit, Alice said that she had recently had trouble breathing and catching her breath. Alice's symptoms were evaluated and it was determined that she had mild emphysema. She was told that she could reduce the chances of the disease getting worse by quitting smoking. Although Alice admitted she enjoyed smoking, especially with her friends, she valued her health. She expressed concern when told that her longevity and ability to function independently as she ages would be in jeopardy if she continued to smoke. Upon learning of the consequences she faced with continued smoking, Alice asked for help in trying to quit. Through physician help, she set a quit date and initiated nicotine fading until she felt she was no longer driven to smoke. Then she applied nicotine patches to control cravings. Social support was recommended which Alice did not think was necessary. However, when slips began to occur, she returned and asked for additional help. The medical education staff showed Alice how to seek and be successful in obtaining social support from family and friends and how to successfully use telephone helplines (e.g., 1–800–4 CANCER) to maintain abstinence. Although she encountered several problems in trying to quit, her persistence led to cessation within a year.

Comment: This case illustrates that a short discussion, personalizing the risks of continued smoking and the rewards of quitting, can lead to immediate action. The key was to make the discussion relevant to the smoker's personal situation. In addition, it shows that even though the smoker received a personalized quit plan, other cessation resources are sometimes needed to address problems as they arise.

Conclusion

Older smokers are a vulnerable group who present a different set of smoking-related circumstances from younger smokers. Specifically, these circumstances include being highly addicted, having smoked for decades, and having health problems that are complicated by smoking, a link that they tend not to understand at first. However, recent research indicates that older smokers are as likely, or more likely, to quit with standard treatments than younger smokers (Orleans, 1997). Nevertheless, successful intervention is not without its barriers. Older smokers are not likely to believe that smoking is hazardous to their health. In addition, they enjoy smoking and consider quitting to be giving up a pleasure that they have grown accustomed to and look forward to. Many fail to see the need for quitting or even want to quit. Convincing this vulnerable group of the risk of continued smoking is a very important step leading to a quit attempt. Research has shown that stage of change-matched treatments produce greater quitting outcomes than stage-mismatched treatments. So, it is important to identify the older smoker's stage of change and apply a treatment suited to that stage. Smoking cessation treatments that emphasize skills development, problem solving, appropriate use of nicotine replacement, and social support are likely to be most effective with this group. Consistent application of tested methods as well as diligent follow-up results in significant smoking cessation outcomes for older smokers.

References

Boyd, N. R., & Orleans, C. T. (1999). Intervening with older smokers. In D. F. Seidman, & L. S. Covey (Editors), *Helping the hard-core smoker: A clinician's guide* (pp. 115–135). Mahwah, NJ: Lawrence Erlbaum Associates.

Centers for Disease Control. (1996). Cigarette smoking among adults—United States, *Morbidity and Mortality Weekly Report, 43,* 588–590.

Cummings, S. R., Rubin, S. M., & Oster, G. (1988). The cost-effectiveness of counseling smokers to quit. *Journal of the American Medical Association, 261,* 75–79.

Fiore, M. C., Bailey, W. C., Cohen, S. J., et al. (1996). *Smoking cessation. Clinical Guideline No. 18.* AHCPR Publication No. 96–0692. Rockville, MD: U.S. Department of Health and Human Services, Public Health Service, Agency for Health Care Policy and Research.

Fiore, M. C., Bailey, W. C., & Cohen, S. J. (2000). *Treating tobacco use and dependence: A clinical practice guideline.* Rockville, MD: U.S. Department of Health and Human Services, Agency for Healthcare Research and Quality Publication No. 00–0032.

Fiore, M., Smith, S. S., Jornby, D. E., & Baker, T. B. (1994). The effectiveness of the nicotine patch for smoking cessation: A meta-analysis. *Journal of the American Medical Association, 271,* 1940–1947.

Fries, J. F., Green, L. W., & Levine, S. (1989). Health promotion and the compression of morbidity. *Lancet, 1,* 481–483.

Glynn, T. J. (1988). Relative effectiveness of physician-initiated smoking cessation programs. *Cancer Bulletin, 40,* 359–364.

Glynn, T. J., & Manley, M. (1990). *How to help your patients stop smoking: A National Cancer Institute manual for physicians.* NIH Publication No. 90–3064. Bethesda, MD: United States Department of Health and Human Services, Public Health Service, National Institutes of Health, National Cancer Institute.

Hurt, R. D., Sachs, D. P. L., Glover, E. D., Offord, K. P., Johnston, J. A., Dale, L. C., Khayrallah, M. A., Schroeder, D. R., Glover, P. N., Sullivan, C. R., Groghan, I. T., & Sullivan, P. M. (1997). A comparison of sustained-release bupropion and placebo for smoking cessation. *New England Journal of Medicine, 33,* 1195–1202.

Krumholz, H. M., Cohen, B. J., Tsevar, J., Pasternak, R. C., & Weinstein, M. C. (1993). Cost-effectivness of a smoking cessation program after myocardial infarction. *American Journal of Cardiology, 22,* 1697–1702.

Lipman, A. G. (1985). How smoking interferes with drug therapy. *Modern Medicine, 8,* 141–142.

Morgan, G. D., Noll, E. L., Orleans, C. T., Rimer, B. K., Amfoh, K., & Bonney, G. (1996). Reaching midlife and older smokers: Tailored interventions for routine medical care. *Preventive Medicine, 25,* 346–354.

Moore, S. R. (1986). Smoking and drug effects in geriatric patients. *Pharmacy International, 7*(1), 1–3.

Orleans, C. T. (1997). Reducing tobacco harms among older adults: A critical agenda for tobacco control. *Tobacco Control, 6,* 161–163.

Orleans, C. T., Jepson, C., Resch, N., & Rimer, B. K. (1994). Quitting motives and barriers among older smokers: The 1986 adult use of tobacco survey revisited, *Cancer, 74,* 2055–2061.

Orleans, C. T., Resch, N., Noll, E., Keintz, M. K., Rimer, B. K., Brown, T. V., & Snedden, T. M. (1994). Use of transdermal nicotine in a statewide prescription plan for the elderly: A first look at "real world" patch users. *Journal of the American Medical Association, 271,* 601–607.

Prochaska, J. O., & DiClemente, C. C. (1983). Stages and processes of self-change of smoking: Toward an integrative model. *Journal of Consulting and Clinical Psychology, 51,* 390–395.

Prochaska, J. O., DiCemente, C. C., Velicer, W. F., & Rossi, J. S. (1993). Standardized, individualized, interactive and personalized self-help programs for smoking cessation. *Health Psychology, 12,* 399–405.

Rimer, B. K., & Orleans, C. T. (1990). Family physicians should intervene with older smokers. *American Family Physician, 42*(4), 959–965.

Rimer, B. K., & Orleans, C. T. (1993). Older smokers. In C. T. Orleans, & J. Slade (Editors). *Nicotine addiction: Principles and management* (pp. 385–395). New York: Oxford University Press.

Rimer, B. K., Orleans, C. T., Fleisher, L., Cristinzios, S., Resche, N., Telepchak, J., & Keintz, M. K. (1994). Does tailoring matter: The impact of a tailored guide on ratings and short-term smoking-related outcomes for older smokers. *Health Education Research, 9*(1), 69–84.

Rimer, B. K., Orleans, C. T., Keintz, M. K., Cristinzio, S., & Fleisher, L. (1990). The older smoker: Status, challenges and opportunities for intervention. *Chest, 97,* 547–553.

Schneider, N. G. (1987). Nicotine gum in smoking cessation: Rationale, efficacy, and proper use. *Comprehensive Therapy, 13,* 32–37.

Shopland, D. R., & Burns, D. M. (1993). Medical and public health implications of tobacco addiction. In C. T. Orleans, & J. Slade, (Editors), *Nicotine addiction: Principles and management* (pp. 105–128). New York: Oxford University Press.

Shopland, D. R., Hartman, A. M., Gibson, J. T., Mueller, M. D., Kessler, L. G., & Lynn, W. R. (1996). Cigarette smoking among U.S. adults by state and region: Estimates from the current population survey. *Journal of the National Cancer Institute, 88,* 1748–1758.

Silagy, C., Mant, D., Fowler, G., & Lodge, M. (1994). Meta-analysis on efficacy of nicotine replacement therapies in smoking cessation. *Lancet, 343,* 139–142.

U.S. Department of Health, Education and Welfare. (1964). *Smoking and health.* Report of the Advisory Committee to the Surgeon General of the Public Health Service. U.S. Department of Health, Education, and Welfare, Public Health Service, Center for Disease Control, PHS Publication No. 1103.

U.S. Department of Health and Human Services. (1990). *Health benefits of smoking cessation: A report of the surgeon general.* (DHHS Publication No. CSC 90-8416) U.S. Department of Health and Human Services & Public Health Service.

Ventura, S. J., Anderson, R. N., Martin, J. A., & Smith, B. L. (1998). Births and deaths: Preliminary data for 1997. *National Statistics Reports, 47,* 4.

Resources: Smoking Cessation Self-Help Guides

Title	Source
Clear Horizons (Only guide designed for older smokers)	Fox Chase Cancer Center 7701 Burholme Avenue Philadelphia, Pennsylvania 19111 1–215–728–3139
Clearing the Air	Office of Cancer Communication National Cancer Institute 9000 Rockville Pike Building 31 Bethesda, Maryland 20892 1–800–4–CANCER
Free and Clear	Center for Health Promotion Group Health Cooperative of Puget Sound Seattle, Washington 98121 1–800–292–2336
Freedom From Smoking for You and Your Family	American Lung Association 1740 Broadway New York, NY 10019 1–212–315–8700

11

Problem Gambling Among Older People

Ronald M. Pavalko

Introduction

This chapter will focus on identifying and treating gambling addiction among older people. First, I will describe what problem gambling is and how prevalent it is. Then I will discuss how the disorder develops, and finally how it is treated.

Definitions: Pathological and Problem Gambling

"Pathological," "compulsive," and "disordered" gambling refer to gambling that meets at least 5 of the American Psychiatric Association's 10 criteria for *pathological gambling* which are presented in Table 11.1.

The term "problem gambling" is used in two ways: 1) to refer to gambling where people develop significant family, work, or financial problems as a consequence of their gambling but do not exhibit the extreme characteristics of pathological gambling; and 2), as a general term, to refer to gambling that adversely affects a person's life to any degree, from mild problems to pathological gambling. This chapter will use the term "problem gambling" in the second, more inclusive, sense, except when quoting or paraphrasing writing that uses other terms.

Table 11.1 The American Psychiatric Association's Diagnostic Criteria for Pathological Gambling (DSM-IV)

1. Preoccupied with gambling (e.g., preoccupied with reliving past gambling experiences, handicapping, or planning the next venture, or thinking of ways to get money with which to gamble).
2. Needs to gamble with increasing amounts of money in order to achieve the desired excitement.
3. Restlessness or irritability when attempting to cut down or stop gambling.
4. Gambles as a way of escaping from problems or relieving dysphoric mood (e.g., feelings of helplessness, guilt, anxiety, or depression).
5. After losing money gambling, often returns another day in order to get even ("chasing" one's losses).
6. Lies to family members or others to conceal the extent of involvement with gambling.
7. Illegal acts (e.g., forgery, fraud, theft, embezzlement) are committed to finance gambling.
8. Has jeopardized or lost significant relationship, job, or educational or career opportunities because of gambling.
9. Reliance on others to provide money to relieve a desperate financial situation caused by gambling (a bailout).
10. Repeated unsuccessful efforts to control, cut back, or stop gambling.

Note. From *Diagnostic and Statistical Manual of Mental Disorders* (4th ed.). 1994. Washington, DC: American Psychiatric Association. Reprinted with permission.

What is Problem Gambling?

Since the early 1970s, research and clinical experience have produced a fairly clear picture of problem gambling that fits an "illness model." Problem gambling has become "medicalized" in the sense that it is defined as a disease that is essentially an addiction. Robert Custer, a pioneer in the treatment of problem gambling, defined it as "an addictive illness" in which the subject is driven by an overwhelming, uncontrollable impulse to gamble. The impulse progresses in intensity and urgency, consuming more and more of the individual's time, energy, and emotional and material resources. Ultimately, it invades, undermines, and often destroys everything that is meaningful in his life" (Custer & Milt, 1985).

Others have described it as "a progressive disorder characterized by a continuous or periodic loss of control over gambling; a preoccupation with gambling and with obtaining money with which to gamble; irrational thinking; and a continuation of the behavior despite adverse consequences" (Rosenthal & Lesieur, 1992).

Basic Characteristics of Problem Gambling

Problem gamblers have an intense *preoccupation* with gambling to the point where it dominates their lives. They gamble more frequently and with more money than they intend to spend, and they cannot control the amount of money or time spent gambling (Lesieur, 1984, 1993; Rosenthal, 1989). Case study #1 illustrates this feature of problem gambling rather well.

Case 1: Hooked on Bingo. In her early 60s when her husband Phil retired, Lena was looking forward to "doing things." But Phil, whom she described as a "couch potato," had other ideas. Watching TV and napping were his ideas of the good life.

When some friends suggested she go with them to play bingo at a local church, she jumped at the chance to get out. Bingo was fun, and an escape from boredom. At first she won a little money, but before long she was losing more than winning. The weekly game turned into a twice-a-week game, and soon she was going to every game she could find, often to several a day.

Lena and Phil had limited financial resources and soon acquiring money for gambling became a problem. While credit card solicitations are viewed by most people as a nuisance, Lena welcomed them. In addition to "maxing out" the credit line on about a dozen cards, she got a home equity loan on the home. Oblivious to what she was doing, Phil would "sign anything I put in front of him."

She reached a point where she had about $100,000 in credit card and home equity loan payments due and no way to pay them. Lena had a part-time job as an accountant at a construction company. She "borrowed" (i.e., embezzled) $75,000, was caught, and arrested. She pleaded guilty and faced a 10-year jail sentence.

Her lawyer sent her to Gamblers Anonymous, hoping to convince the court that she recognized the seriousness of her addiction and was doing something about it. It worked. She got a suspended sentence with 10 years' probation. A plan for repaying the construction company was worked out.

When I met Lena she had been "clean" for a little over 3 years. She was participating in individual counseling and regularly attending GA meetings. She also spends a good deal of time now talking to older people about the addiction potential of gambling.

Case 2: No Easy Solution. Bill had been a gambler and salesman all his life. His gambling involved betting on horse races and sporting events, with an occasional trip to a casino. His gambling usually involved small amounts of money well within his budget. That changed when his wife died at the age of 64.

Bill, 67 at the time of his wife's death, found himself alone, depressed, and looking at an unknown future. Still working in sales, he was "on the road" a good deal, working with minimal supervision. Continuing to make bets through his bookie, he also spent an increasing amount of time at racetracks and casinos throughout the upper Midwest as he traveled on his job. Gambling was a great escape for him and before long the job was secondary to gambling.

Within a year, Bill had gone through about $150,000, his total life savings. At one point he owed his bookie about $20,000. Bill learned about GA after calling an "800 Helpline" number posted at a riverboat casino in Illinois. He began attending meetings, entered group counseling with a certified gambling counselor, and had been in recovery about 3 years when I met him.

Over the next 5 years Bill tried gambling in a "controlled" way. It didn't work. He dropped out of GA and the counseling group and began spending more and more time at casinos. During these 5 years he was in and out of GA at least three times. The last I heard (about 2 years ago) he was gambling again. He knows he has a problem but just can't deal with it. Whether he will ever fully cope with his addiction is uncertain.

Problem gamblers develop a pattern analogous to what in other addictions is called *tolerance.* The amount of money they bet increases and they move from simple bets to those where the risks and the potential winnings are greater, as illustrated by Bill in Case Study #2. They also exhibit symptoms analogous to *withdrawal* symptoms, when they try to cut back or stop gambling, can't get to a gambling venue, or do not have money with which to gamble (McGowan & Chamberlain, 2000; Pavalko, 2000). In these circumstances they exhibit irritability, nervousness, restlessness, and anger. The most important thing that distinguishes problem gamblers from recreational gamblers is *chasing.* Compulsive gamblers "chase" their losses, that is, they continue betting in the face of mounting losses, trying to get even or win back what they have lost (Lesieur, 1984). They also live in a world of secrecy and deceit. They try to keep their gambling a secret as long as possible by *lying to family and friends* about their gambling activities, losses, and debts. They become very skilled at doing this. As long as they can keep others from discovering their problem, they can deny its existence to themselves as well.

When financial problems become severe, or when the gamblers run out of ways to borrow money, problem gamblers may engage in *illegal activities* to obtain money with which to gamble or to pay off their debts. Engaging in crime is often a matter of convenience and opportunity. Access to an employer's funds or a client's account may be seen as an easy way to solve their financial problems. Embezzlement, forgery, misappropriation of funds, and tax and insurance fraud are the most common crimes committed by problem gamblers. Clearly, Lena, in case study #1, took advantage of this kind of opportunity. Crimes like robbery, burglary, shoplifting, and drug dealing also occur, but less frequently. Elderly problem gamblers are probably less likely than younger people to engage in these kinds of criminal activity.

Problem gamblers have a high incidence of insomnia, intestinal disorders, migraine headaches, and other stress-related disorders, and depression is quite common (McGowan & Chamberlain, 2000; Pavalko, 2000). Whether they gamble to relieve depression (as the DSM-IV criteria suggest) or whether depression is a result of their gambling (indebtedness, marital conflicts, job loss) is an unresolved issue. Members of Gamblers Anonymous (GA) have a high attempted suicide rate—about six times higher than the general population. One study of 162 GA members found that 13 percent had attempted suicide and 21 percent had given it serious consideration (Frank, Lester, & Wexler, 1991).

Personality and Other Characteristics of Problem Gamblers

While there is not a distinctive "problem gambler personality type," problem gamblers do exhibit some common personality characteristics. Not every problem gambler will exhibit all of them or exhibit them to the same degree, since there is a great deal of variation among problem gamblers. Some are "action seekers," drawn to gambling for the excitement it offers. Others are "escape gamblers" who use gambling as an escape from a variety of personal problems.

Problem gamblers tend to be very intelligent, energetic, hard-working people who enjoy challenging tasks such as handicapping races or sporting events, or learning the decision rules of blackjack (Lesieur, 1984; Pavalko, 2000). They also tend to be narcissistic, arrogant, and very self-confident (Lesieur, 1984, 1993; Rosenthal, 1989). They are apt to believe that they are exempt from the laws of probability that apply to everyone else.

Problem gamblers also have a tendency to try to control events. Gambling provides the illusion that they can control the uncontrollable. Their thinking can become so irrational that they believe they can control the turn of a card, the roll of the dice, or the outcome of a race. In the advanced stages of this disorder, cause and effect become reversed. Instead of seeing their financial, family, work, legal, and other problems as the *result* of their gambling, they see additional gambling as the *solution* to those problems.

Cross Addiction and Addiction Switching

Chemical dependency and problem gambling clearly are related. About half of the GA members and problem gamblers in treatment report a serious chemical addiction (usually alcohol) at some point in their lives and for long periods of time. About 20 percent of people receiving inpatient treatment for chemical dependency are problem gamblers (Pavalko, 2000). A recent study of 1,051 patients seeking help for medical problems (but not for gambling) at three primary-care Wisconsin clinics found a relationship between problem gambling and chemical use. Compared with patients who did not have a gambling problem, problem gamblers were more likely to be heavy users of alcohol and marijuana, and to smoke cigarettes (Pasternak & Fleming, 1999).

Addiction "switching" also occurs. Counselors report that about 10 percent of recovering alcoholics replace their alcohol use with gambling, and about the same proportion of recovering problem gamblers develop alcohol problems (Blume, 1994).

Unfortunately, we do not know whether cross-addiction and addiction switching are age related. Similarly, there are no published studies on how the basic characteristics of problem gambling and the personality characteristics of problem gamblers may vary by age.

Differences Between Problem Gambling and Chemical Addiction

While problem gambling is similar to chemical addiction, there are some important differences. Problem gamblers do not ingest, inject, or inhale substances like chemically addicted people do. This raises the crucial question of just what they become addicted to. When problem gamblers are asked about this, the answer they give is "action," an aroused, euphoric state involving excitement, tension, and anticipation of the outcome of a gambling event. It is the thrill of living "on the edge." Problem gamblers describe action as a "high," using language similar to that used by chemically addicted people. Some experience these sensations just thinking about gambling as well as when they are actually gambling. Action also has been described as a "rush" that may include rapid heartbeat, sweaty palms, and nausea. Problem gamblers routinely describe being in action as "better than drugs and better than sex." When in action, they lose track of time; sleep, food, water or using a bathroom take a backseat to staying in action.

Addiction to an activity rather than a substance is much more difficult to explain in terms of basic biological mechanisms, and more difficult to detect (and easier to conceal from friends, family members, and counselors) because of the absence of physical signs. This is why problem gambling is often referred to as a "hidden addiction" (Pavalko, 1999).

Another difference from chemical addiction lies in the ability of problem gamblers to pursue their addiction as long as they have the financial resources to do so. It is impossible to "overdose" on gambling the way one can overdose on alcohol or other drugs. While alcoholics or people addicted to other drugs can consume their drug to the point where they do severe physical damage to themselves, problem gamblers can continue gambling without such consequences. The concept of overdosing simply has no counterpart in gambling addiction.

Problem gambling is also viewed differently from chemical addiction by counselors, the human services system, and society at large. Until very recently counselors who encountered problem gamblers for *other* problems have not been well informed about this disorder. Problem gambling has not been a topic routinely covered in the professional education of counselors, and very few public or private human service agencies have had gambling treatment experts on staff. Hardly any members of GA report that they were referred to the organization by a mental health professional. Members of GA treated by psychiatrists, psychologists, and counselors for other problems are rarely asked about their gambling behavior. The health insurance industry also treats problem gambling differently from the way it treats chemical addiction; in the United States there is no health insurance coverage for a *primary* diagnosis of "pathological" gambling, even though it is included in the DSM-IV. The Americans With Disabilities Act specifically excludes gambling addicts from its coverage, while it includes substance addicts.

There is also a low level of public understanding of problem gambling as an addiction and a disorder. All too often, many people regard the problem gambler as just a bad, stupid, or irresponsible person. During at least the past 50 years, the medical profession, the mass media, and self-help groups have slowly developed an awareness among the general public that alcoholism and addiction to other drugs are diseases. Efforts to redefine problem gambling as a "real" disorder are still in their infancy.

Participation of Older People in Gambling

Although our focus is on the elderly, we need a benchmark or baseline for looking at both their participation in gambling and the prevalence of their problem gambling. Do they gamble more or less than younger people? How has the gambling behavior of older people changed over time?

Research on gambling participation typically uses two measures: "past-year gambling" (whether one has gambled during the year preceding the study) and "lifetime gambling" (whether one has ever gambled).

State surveys conducted during the early 1990s report *lifetime* gambling rates ranging from a low of 72 percent in Georgia to a high of 92 percent in New Jersey, with Texas at 76 percent. Surveys in Wisconsin and Nebraska report *past-year* gambling rates of 66 and 62 percent, respectively (summarized in Pavalko, 2000).

In 1998 the National Opinion Research Center (NORC) conducted a survey for the National Gambling Impact Study Commission (NGISC). It collected data from a national sample of adults on gambling participation. A commission like NGISC collected similar data in 1975, making it possible to look at changes in gambling rates over time. For all ages grouped together, *past-year* gambling essentially held steady, increasing from 61 to 63 percent. However, *lifetime* gambling increased from 68 to 86 percent (National Opinion Research Center et al., 1999).

How do the elderly compare with younger people? In 1975, people 65 and older had a *lifetime* gambling participation rate of only 35%, compared with a rate of 67% of those in the 45–64 age group, 74% for those age 25–44, and 75% for those age 18–24. By 1998, the elderly had caught up to younger people. Their lifetime gambling participation rate of 80% was identical to that of people age 18–24, and only 8 percentage points lower than those in the two intermediate age groups (National Opinion Research Center et al., 1999). This is a striking, dramatic indicator of increased participation in gambling by the elderly.

Past-year gambling participation by the elderly has also undergone a significant change, albeit less dramatic than for lifetime participation. In 1975, 23% of those 65 and over had gambled during the past year, compared with 60% of those age 45–64, 69% of those age 25–44, and 73% of those age 18–24. By 1998, the elderly had closed the gap considerably. Fifty percent had gambled during the past year, compared to the younger age groups which ranged from 64% to 67% (National Opinion Research Center et al., 1999).

The gambling gender gap also is closing. In 1975, 61% of women had gambled at some time in their lives compared with 75% of men. By 1998, the figure was up to 83% for women, compared with 88% for men. A similar pattern exists for *past-year* gambling. Between 1975 and 1998, the percentage of past-year female gamblers rose from 55% to 60% while the rate for men held steady (68% versus 67%) (National Opinion Research Center et al., 1999).

The Prevalence of Problem Gambling

How prevalent is problem gambling? Since the mid-1980s numerous surveys have been conducted throughout the United States. When the findings of these surveys are averaged, the result is that about 4.4% of the adult population are problem gamblers (for a more detailed analysis of these surveys, see Pavalko, 2000).

In a review of 120 prevalence studies, Shaffer and associates (1997) concluded that gamblers who meet the DSM-IV criteria for pathological gambling constitute 1.60% of the general adult population and that an additional 3.85% are gamblers for whom gambling has created a variety of problems (Shaffer, Hall, & Vander Bilt, 1997).

The NORC study noted earlier included interviews with a random sample of 2,417 adults and 530 patrons at gambling facilities. It estimated that approximately 1.2% of the adult population (about 2.5 million people) met the DSM-IV criteria for "pathological gambling" and that an additional 1.5% (about 3 million people) were "problem gamblers." A variety of research, including estimates done before and after the introduction of new forms of gambling, supports the conclusion that the more available gambling is, the higher the prevalence of problem gambling (Pavalko, 2000; Shaffer et al., 1997).

Age and Prevalence of Problem Gambling

The best data on the relationship between age and the prevalence of problem gambling come from the survey done in 1998 by NORC for the NGISC. These data are presented in Table 11.2. A screening instrument developed specifically for this survey was based on the DSM-IV criteria for pathological gambling. In Table 11.2, "at risk" gamblers are people who met one or two of the DSM-IV criteria; "problem" gamblers are those who met three or four criteria; and "pathological" gamblers are those who met five or more criteria.

As expected, lifetime rates for all levels of gambling problems and all age groups are higher than past-year rates. While the relationship is not a perfect one, it is generally the case that prevalence rates decrease as age increases, a finding consistent with the results of earlier research at the state level. Several things stand out regarding people age 65 and older. First, the proportion of at-risk gamblers (lifetime rate) among those 65 and older is the same as for those age 50–64. Second, the

Table 11.2 Lifetime and Past-Year Prevalence of Gambling Problems, by Age, in Percentages

	At Risk (*N*=267) Life/Year		Problem (*N*=56) Life/Year		Pathological (*N*=67) Life/Year	
Age						
18–29	10.1	3.9	2.1	1.0	1.3	0.3
30–39	6.9	2.1	1.5	0.8	1.0	0.6
40–49	8.9	3.3	1.9	0.7	1.4	0.8
50–64	6.1	3.6	1.2	0.3	2.2	0.9
65+	6.1	1.7	0.7	0.6	0.4	0.2

Note. From *Gambling Impact and Behavior Study: Report to the National Gambling Impact Study Commission,* National Opinion Research Center, Gemini Research, The Lewin Group, and Christiansen/Cummings Associates, www.norc.uchicago.edu, downloaded April 1, 1999, Table 7, pp. 26 and 27. Reprinted with permission.

proportion of problem gamblers (past-year rate) is higher among those 65 and older than for those age 50–64. And among those with the most serious gambling problems (i.e., pathological) during the past year, persons 65 and older more closely resemble the 18–29 age group than the intermediate age groups, all of which had higher rates.

Prevalence rates for the elderly are not available for men and women separately, but other data in the NORC survey are suggestive of the dynamics of the development of gambling problems. Prevalence rates for men are consistently higher than those for women. This is in all likelihood due to the fact that women are relative newcomers to commercial gambling. There is also an interesting relationship between marital status and some prevalence rates. Widowed people have a higher past year at-risk gambling rate than married or cohabiting people, but a lower rate than divorced, separated, or never married people (National Opinion Research Center, et al., 1999; pp. 26–27). While widowed people are found in all age groups, they are more likely to be found among those over 65, suggesting that, as many counselors report, widowhood may play a role in the development of at least some gambling problems among the elderly.

Problem Gambling Careers

The development of problem gambling usually follows a typical sequence, originally identified by Custer and Milt (1985). The sequence includes three stages: winning, losing, and desperation. In the *winning phase* occasional gambling often includes frequent wins and is accompanied by increased excitement, more frequent gambling, and increased amounts of money being wagered. The early careers of problem gamblers usually include a "big win," although it tends to occur more often among action-seeking gamblers than among "escape" gamblers. When it does occur, the big win creates unreasonable optimism and fantasies about continuing to win big. The big win also serves as a "baseline" for the future. As losses inevitably occur, the gambler "knows" he or she can win big again because it has happened before. The winning phase also includes bragging about how much one is winning, thinking about gambling to the exclusion of other things, and a feeling of being invulnerable.

Wins cannot continue indefinitely. It is inherent in the basic structure of commercial gambling (especially casino games) that the laws of probability and the house advantage built into the games will inevitably result in losses. As gamblers enter the *losing phase,* there are prolonged losing episodes in which they chase losses, remain confident that a big win is just around the corner, and simply cannot stop gambling. The gamblers profiled in both case studies illustrate this sequence. They begin borrowing from friends, relatives, banks (second mortgages, personal loans), and take credit card advances, and markers (short-term loans) from casinos. Gamblers neglect family responsibilities, delay paying bills, lose time from work, and lie about their gambling and their losses. Personality changes, including irritability, restlessness, and depression occur. Older gamblers are likely to spend their Social Security and other annuity income, exhaust their savings, and cash in their investments.

Gamblers enter the *desperation phase* as their ability to pay bills and loans becomes more difficult. Their borrowing becomes heavier and they may turn to loan sharks and bookies. They become increasingly alienated from friends and family who, having been "burned" many times, refuse to bail them out. Toward the end of this phase, gambling becomes more frantic and gambling-related problems dominate the gambler's life. At this point they may commit crimes to get money. They begin blaming others for their problems (especially those who won't loan them money), which exacerbates their alienation and isolation. Hopelessness, suicidal thoughts and attempts, arrest, divorce, alcohol problems, emotional breakdowns, and gambling-related withdrawal symptoms all can be part of the end of the desperation phase.

This scenario is a generalized pattern. The careers of particular individuals may not involve all the steps included in each phase and the rate at which they move through each phase can vary.

There is no reason to think that this general pattern does not occur in elderly people. However, some parts of the pattern may be different for some older adults. To the extent that the elderly lack friends or relatives to borrow money from, the amount and extent of borrowing among older people may be less than for younger people. The work-related difficulties naturally are not relevant for people who are retired, and retired people would not be in a position to commit work-related "white collar" crimes, although forgery and tax and insurance fraud would still be possibilities. They also would probably be less likely to engage in other types of crime to get money.

Triggers and At-Risk Factors Among the Elderly

There are several features of the lives of older people that make the development of gambling problems somewhat different from the way these problems develop among younger people. It is useful to think of these as "triggers" or special predisposing factors.

One important factor is *opportunity*. Regardless of where they live, legal gambling is more readily available to elderly people today than it was in the past. When legal gambling was limited to Nevada and Atlantic City, getting to a gambling venue was an elaborate and costly undertaking. With the recent growth of gambling, racinos (race tracks with casinos), riverboats, and Native American casinos are a short drive or a low-cost, often subsidized, bus ride away, and older people have the time to participate.

The "sunbelt" states, to which many older people have retired, provide ample gambling opportunities. Arizona and California both have Native American reservation casinos, and their proximity to Nevada makes for easy access to the world's premier gambling destination, Las Vegas. In Florida, elderly retirees have horse and dog racing, JaiAlai, Native American reservation casinos, and a concentration of gambling "cruises to nowhere." Nationally, nearly $3.9 billion was wagered in 1998 on casino boats that provide gambling once they are in international waters (Christiansen, 1999).

Boredom is also a trigger that leads many older people to gamble. Gambling is a way of filling the abundant leisure time that many older people experience following retirement. Older people with physical limitations may be limited in the kinds of activities in which they can engage. Gambling is a relatively passive leisure activity. Many casinos now provide "handicapped only" blackjack tables that accommodate wheelchairs.

For older people experiencing *loneliness* or *isolation* as a result of the loss of a spouse or close friends, gambling is a way of being in proximity to, if not interacting with, other people. The death of his wife was clearly a trigger that propelled Bill (in Case Study #2) into uncontrolled gambling. Gambling venues, especially casinos, are exciting, fun places. Getting out and being around other people can be a powerful stimulus to engage in gambling. Gambling may give people the feeling of being part of something rather than being alone. Ironically, playing slot machines, which is popular among older people, can be a very isolated activity.

But, to the extent that it provides a diversion from routines, gambling can have a great appeal to older people. Just how appealing it is can be seen in the results of a recent survey of 6,957 Nebraskans 65 and older. Twenty-three percent reported playing bingo more than four times a month and 16% took day trips to casinos more than once a month. They were more likely to engage in these gambling activities than to take trips to museums, libraries, or zoos, pursue hobbies, or go to restaurants (McNeilly & Burke, 1998).

Gambling is a marvelous *escape*. It is a fantasy world in which one can leave behind whatever problems one may want to forget about—poor health, loss of a spouse, distant grandchildren. In both case studies (but especially for Bill in #2), gambling was an escape. Casinos in particular facilitate the creation of a fantasy world. It is no accident that clocks and windows are hard to find in them, and that night turns into day. Initially at least, gambling for many older people may be an effective solution to whatever problems they are trying to escape from.

The *gambling industry's marketing practices* also contribute to a high rate of gambling among older people. They are a "target market." Free admission to race tracks and free or low-cost transportation to casinos are among the many promotions used to attract older customers. "Comps" (complimentary meals, lodging, gifts) are widely used. Casino operators have also developed hospitality programs that emphasize making older people feel welcome and that cater to their interests and needs.

Assessment for Problem Gambling

There are a number of tools available for the assessment of problem gambling in a clinical setting. The *DSM-IV criteria* are one important assessment tool. Diagnosis involves a clinician reaching a conclusion based on information obtained directly from a client supplemented, if possible, by information from family, friends, or other treatment professionals. If a person exhibits five or more of the behaviors included in the criteria, he or she should be considered to be a "pathological gambler." Of course, a person meeting one to four of the criteria may have a problem without scoring at the "pathological" level.

Another instrument used to identify problem gambling is the *Gamblers Anonymous 20 Questions,* presented in Table 11.3. It can be self-administered or used in an interview. A person answering "yes" to seven

Table 11.3 Gamblers Anonymous 20 Questions

1. Did you ever lose time from work due to gambling?
2. Has gambling ever made your home life unhappy?
3. Did gambling affect your reputation?
4. Have you ever felt remorse after gambling?
5. Did you ever gamble to get money with which to pay debts or otherwise solve financial difficulties?
6. Did gambling cause a decrease in your ambition or efficiency?
7. After losing did you feel you must return as soon as possible and win back your losses?
8. After a win did you have a strong urge to return and win more?
9. Did you often gamble until your last dollar was gone?
10. Did you ever borrow to finance your gambling?
11. Have you ever sold any real or personal property to finance gambling?
12. Were you reluctant to use "gambling money" for normal expenditures?
13. Did gambling make you careless of the welfare of your family?
14. Did you ever gamble longer than you had planned?
15. Have you ever gambled to escape worry or trouble?
16. Have you ever committed, or considered committing, an illegal act to finance gambling?
17. Did gambling cause you to have difficulty in sleeping?
18. Do arguments, disappointments, or frustrations create within you an urge to gamble?
19. Did you ever have an urge to celebrate any good fortune by a few hours of gambling?
20. Have you ever considered self-destruction as a result of your gambling?

Note. Gamblers Anonymous, P.O. Box 17173, Los Angeles, CA 90017. Reprinted with permission.

or more of the questions should be considered to be a compulsive gambler. Like the DSM-IV criteria, fewer than seven "yes" answers does not necessarily mean that the person has no gambling problem.

In the mid-1980s a sociologist and a psychiatrist developed the *South Oaks Gambling Screen (SOGS).* Revised in 1993 (Lesieur & Blume, 1993), it has until quite recently been the primary tool used in the identification of problem gambling in both clinical settings and in survey research. It includes 20 scored questions, many of which are similar to the DSM-IV criteria and GA's 20 Questions. The questions measure such behaviors as concealing evidence of gambling, gambling longer and with more money than intended, and arguing with family members over gambling and borrowing. A score of five or more indicates a "probable pathological gambler" and a score of one to four indicates "some problem" with gambling. Space limitations preclude reproducing the instrument here. It is available from two sources: Lesieur and Blume (1993) and Pavalko (2000).

A final assessment instrument is the *National Opinion Research Center/DSM-IV Screen (NODS).* The NODS was specifically developed to closely reflect the DSM-IV criteria. It measures preoccupation with gambling, tolerance, withdrawal, loss of control, use of gambling to escape from problems, chasing losses, lying, committing illegal acts, risking significant relationships, and bailouts. In all likelihood the NODS will replace the SOGS in survey research to estimate problem-gambling prevalence rates in large populations.

One positive feature of the NODS is that it identifies *degrees* of a gambling problem by distinguishing among low-risk, at-risk, problem, and pathological gamblers. This instrument also is too long to reproduce here. It is available from two sources: the NGISC report (1999) and the NORC study website (www.norc.uchicago. edu).

No screening instruments have been developed for use specifically with the elderly and none of these instruments has a "senior" version. All the instruments ask about whether gambling interferes with work, an issue that would be irrelevant to retired people. The instruments also ask about the impact of gambling on family members, especially spouses, again, a question obviously irrelevant for older, widowed people. Since a few questions in these instruments do not apply to some older people, one needs to be aware of these difficulties when interpreting the results.

The Treatment of Problem Gambling Among the Elderly

The treatment of problem gambling should be assigned to counselors with specific training (and ideally certification) in dealing with this disorder. Appropriate training consists of completion of the National Council on Problem Gambling's (NCPG) National Gambling Counselor Training Program. The NCPG's Certification Program involves completion of the training program and 2000 hours of supervised counseling of problem gamblers. Many of the 33 (as of January, 1999) state councils on problem gambling and the Canadian Foundation on Compulsive Gambling also provide gambling-specific counselor training.

While problem gamblers should be referred to a qualified counselor, other counselors and providers serving the elderly in many roles may encounter people with a gambling problem and be in a position to provide assistance, information, and referral.

Regardless of age, there are a number of issues and principles involved in the treatment of problem gambling. The following section will review these and identify issues unique to the elderly. The two case studies from the author's files presented earlier will be used to illustrate some of these issues.

Issues Affecting Entry Into Treatment: Denial, Shame, and Resentment

For all problem gamblers, *denial* is a major obstacle to getting help. Once gambling becomes the main activity in a person's life, giving it up may mean giving up one of the few things in life that has any meaning. Seeking help also means confronting the fact that one's fantasies about big wins are nothing more than fantasies. Counselors experienced in treating both problem gamblers and alcoholics say that denial is much stronger among the former.

While all problem gamblers are likely to be ashamed of the trouble they have gotten into with gambling, *shame* may be more pronounced among older people and serve as an obstacle to admitting that a problem exists and to getting help. Age and wisdom supposedly go together. By the time a person reaches his or her 60s, one is supposed to "know better" than to have gambled away one's money. Admitting this to family members, especially one's children, can be extremely painful and may be avoided at all costs by pretending that the problem doesn't exist.

Resentment is an understandable response in older people when anyone questions how they are spending their time and money. Having spent one's life working hard and saving, many older people believe that they have earned the right to spend their time and money as they please. When family members intervene (particularly children) and try to refer an older problem gambler to GA or a counselor, resentment may reach the point where relationships are seriously threatened. Another case illustrates this. In a three-month period following the death of his wife, a 78-year-old problem gambler lost about $75,000 (virtually his life savings). Efforts on the part of his son to link him to GA and other counseling agencies were aggressively rejected with the explanation that the son was only interested in inheriting his father's money.

Entry Into Treatment

Compared with chemical dependence, referral mechanisms for problem-gambling are far less well developed. As already noted, referral by mental health professionals for problem gambling counseling does not occur routinely. There are no legally mandated counseling programs for problem gambling. Problem gambling isn't a crime, unlike illegal drug use, public drunkenness, or drunk driving. Consequently, the legal system does not serve as a useful referral mechanism.

How do people enter treatment for a gambling addiction? The decision to seek help typically occurs when dramatic crises occur, and the gambler feels coerced or "blackmailed" into seeking help.

A spouse or partner may leave or threaten to leave, or file for divorce. A lawyer representing a person arrested for a gambling-related crime may press the client into treatment in an effort to convince a judge or jury that the person has acknowledged the problem and is doing something about it. Having embezzled money from an employer or client, the gambler may seek help to ward off criminal charges. Lena, in Case Study #1, is a good illustration of this. In addition, a bank or loan company may threaten to foreclose. Or a failed suicide attempt may prompt a search for help.

Treatment Goals

An unresolved treatment issue is just what the goal of treatment should be. Some counselors see a complete cessation of gambling as the goal, in effect replacing gambling with "not gambling" as the focal point of the gambler's life. Others see this as a crucial first step, but see the identification and treatment of the underlying problems that led to problem gambling as the real goal.

Whether total abstinence from gambling is essential for successful treatment is another unresolved issue. The vast majority of problem gambling counselors and GAs take this position. However, the possibility that a problem gambler could learn to become a "controlled gambler" has been raised by more than a few researchers and counselors (Dickerson, 1984; Rosecrance, 1988; Schaler, 2000).

Individual Counseling

Treating problem gambling requires efforts to dramatically change the problem gambler's lifestyle and the irrational, fantasy-based way in which gambling is viewed. This may be even more difficult for older problem gamblers who have settled into a "comfortable" lifestyle and may be quick to reject changes of any kind. For many problem gamblers, gambling is a symptom of underlying psychological problems that they are trying to cope with. Treatment may have to address those problems as well as the gambling itself.

There is no single counseling technique for treating problem gambling that a majority of counselors would agree on, except that virtually all agree that, to be effective, individual counseling needs to be combined with participation in GA.

Logically, the treatment of problem gambling should be based on an understanding of its cause. Since the cause is not clearly understood, it is not surprising that no single treatment approach has emerged. Treatment approaches can be grouped into four broad types: aversion therapy, behavioral counseling, desensitization, and cognitive-behavioral therapy. In a review of the effectiveness of these approaches, Lesieur (1998) found mixed results, with no one method proving superior to the others.

Practical Assistance for Problem Gamblers Receiving Treatment

A first step in treatment often is simply *education* about the nature of the disorder. Problem gamblers tend to be confused and bewildered. They see other people gambling without adverse consequences and cannot understand what has happened to them.

Problem gamblers' finances are usually in a state of chaos. They owe money to friends, relatives, credit card issuers, finance companies, loan sharks, bookies, and casinos. They may not have filed income tax returns for some time, and they may be facing foreclosure on home or business mortgages. *Financial advice* from a lawyer or credit counselor may be needed to bring some semblance of order into the problem gambler's financial and legal difficulties. *Legal help* may also be needed to deal with outstanding or imminent criminal charges resulting from bad checks, forgery, embezzlement, tax fraud, or insurance fraud.

It is also essential to develop a *household budget* that may include putting the problem gambler on an allowance, something that the problem gambler can be expected to object to very strongly. Older people are likely to be very hostile to this part of treatment, especially if they have been in control of family finances, or if one or more of their children assumes control of their "allowance." Also essential is developing a "restitution plan" for paying back all the people and organizations from which money has been borrowed. This forces confrontation of the scope of the financial problem and the adverse impact that gambling has had on others.

If employed, it is likely that the problem gambler's job is in jeopardy due to absenteeism, tardiness, and less than conscientious work performance. If this is the case, with the consent of the client, *communication with the employer* about the nature of the employee's problem and the treatment plan is necessary.

If *chemical addiction* is present, treatment will need to confront this problem too. However, it is not appropriate to treat problem gamblers (dually addicted or not) by arranging counseling or entry into self-help groups designed to deal only with chemical addiction.

When depression or other *psychiatric disorders* coexist in problem gamblers, mental health assessment, referral, consultation, and treatment should be arranged.

Family Treatment

Treating problem gambling means treating not just the problem gambler but also family members. At a minimum, this means the spouse and children. In the case of older people it may also mean grandchildren. Family members are likely to be as confused as the gambler about what has been going on. The financial problems of the gambler are also the problems of the spouse. Children, grandchildren, and other relatives may have inadvertently helped the problem gambler by providing loans, alibis, and other bailouts.

Like the problem gambler, family members may have been denying the existence of the problem for a long time. They have been the victims of the problem gambler's lies and deceit. Frustration and resentment are likely to be intense, especially for the spouse and children who have experienced material deprivations as well as emotional distress because of the gambler's conduct. Family members, especially spouses, should be referred to GamAnon, an adjunct of GA.

Table 11.4 Key Components of Successful Treatment

1. In order to avoid the risk of relapse, the problem gambler should avoid exposure to gambling cues and situations, and involvement with other gamblers.
2. Stress-management techniques need to be used to lower arousal and anxiety, and serve as a more appropriate way of coping than gambling.
3. If "dysphoric mood" (especially depression) is experienced, antidepressants may need to be prescribed by a physician.
4. Illogical and erroneous beliefs, attitudes, and expectations regarding gambling need to be challenged and corrected with an emphasis placed on preventing relapse.
5. Marriage/family counseling may be needed to reestablish trust between partners.
6. Budgeting skills and acceptance of financial responsibility need to be developed with a concern for meeting financial obligations without gambling.
7. Developing nongambling leisure activities is essential.
8. If present, addiction to alcohol or other drugs needs to be addressed.
9. Attending Gamblers Anonymous meetings and attending GamAnon meetings by the spouse are essential.

Note. From "Cognitive and Behavioral Therapies for Pathological Gambling," by Alex Blaszczynski, & Derrick Silove, 1995, *Journal of Gambling Studies, 11,* pp. 195–220. Reprinted with permission.

Success in Treatment

Some key components of successful treatment have been identified by Blaszczynski and Silove (1995). They reviewed over a dozen different therapies and identified nine common elements of successful treatment. These are presented in Table 11.4.

However, following these guidelines is no assurance of success. Relapse is very high among problem gamblers, as Bill, in Case Study #2, illustrates. However, these elements represent a core of principles that help maximize the chances of success. It is the therapist's responsibility to make sure that these conditions are being met.

Treatment strategies and programs focused specifically on the elderly have yet to be developed. There is no reason to think that the components of successful treatment outlined in Table 11.4 are not as relevant to the elderly as to younger people.

Gamblers Anonymous

The importance of GA in the treatment of problem gamblers has been noted several times in this chapter. A few comments about GA and its program are in order. GA is a "12-step" self-help recovery program. In many respects, it is modeled after the Alcoholics Anonymous (AA) recovery program. The reason for this is that one of the founders of GA (known as "Jim W.") was also a recovering alcoholic and familiar with the AA program.

Despite similarities between the AA and GA recovery programs, there are some important differences. GA has a different approach to spirituality. Compared with AA, there are fewer direct references to God, and when that word is used it is qualified in various ways. For example, in AA one of the 12 steps is to make "a decision to turn our will and our lives over to the care of God as we understand Him." In GA, one of the steps is "Admitting to ourselves and to another human being the exact nature of our wrongs." In GA, the goal is achieving abstinence from gambling. While GA acknowledges that gambling is a symptom of other problems, there is less concern with addressing those problems than in AA.

Another difference is "consciousness development." While one of the AA steps refers to restoring members to "sanity," GA's comparable step stresses restoring members to a "normal" way of thinking and living. Browne (1991) has pointed out that GA has adapted the AA program by stressing a "secular, medically oriented path" rather than AA's "spiritually oriented path."

While members of both AA and GA see themselves as "deviants," there is a difference in perceptions about how easily they can eliminate the deviant label, be "relabeled," and develop an explanation for their behavior. The alcoholic's behavior is relabeled as a physical illness over which one has no control. This physical illness explanation of alcoholism has become a culturally accepted way of understanding the alcoholic's behavior. In the case of problem gambling, there is no evidence of physical illness or disease, and the idea of the problem gambler as a "sick person" does not enjoy the same degree of cultural acceptance. Consequently, it is more difficult for the problem gambler than the alcoholic to develop a new self-conception that has a shared meaning (Preston & Smith, 1985). Nevertheless, participation in GA, and GamAnon for spouses, is an essential part of the recovery process.

Summary

Gambling among the elderly has clearly increased over the past 25 years as the availability of legal gambling has increased. In its more extreme forms, problem gambling is an addiction similar in many ways to addiction to alcohol and other drugs. The absence of any substance or clear physical signs of problem gambling makes it easy to conceal and difficult to detect, and contributes to its being a hidden addiction. Those who develop this disorder go through distinctive "phases" involving winning, losing, and desperation. A number of assessment tools are available for screening people for problem gambling, but there is no screen specifically for the elderly. In combination with participation in Gamblers Anonymous, a variety of individual and family counseling strategies are used for treating problem gambling.

References

Blaszczynski, A., & Silove, D. (1995). Cognitive and behavioral therapies for pathological gambling. *Journal of Gambling Studies, 11,* 193–220.

Blume, S. B. (1994). Pathological gambling and switching addictions: Report of a case. *Journal of Gambling Studies, 10,* 87–96.

Browne, B. R. (1991). The selective adaptation of the Alcoholics Anonymous program by Gamblers Anonymous. *Journal of Gambling Studies, 7,* 187–206.

Christiansen, E. M. (1999). The 1998 gross annual wager. *International Gaming and Wagering Business, 20,* 17–25.

Custer, R., & Milt, H. (1985). *When luck runs out: Help for compulsive gamblers and their families.* New York: Facts on File Publications.

Dickerson, M. (1984). *Compulsive gamblers.* London: Longman.

Frank, M. L., Lester, D., & Wexler, A. (1991). Suicidal behavior among members of Gamblers Anonymous. *Journal of Gambling Studies, 7,* 249–253.

Lesieur, H. R. (1993). *Understanding compulsive gambling,* Center City, MN: Hazelden Educational Materials.

Lesieur, H. R. (1984). *The chase: Career of the compulsive gambler,* Rochester, VT: Schenkman Books.

Lesieur, H. R. (1998). Cost and treatment of pathological gambling. *The Annals, 556,* 153–169.

Lesieur, H. R., & Blume, S. B. (1993). Revising the South Oaks Gambling Screen in different settings. *Journal of Gambling Studies, 9,* 213–219.

McGowan, W. G., & Chamberlain, L. L. (2000). *Best possible odds: Contemporary treatment strategies for gambling disorders.* New York: John Wiley & Sons.

McNeilly, D. P., & Burke, W. J. (1998). Gambling as a social activity of older adults. Paper presented at the 12th National Conference on Problem Gambling, Las Vegas, NV.

National Opinion Research Center, Gemini Research, The Lewin Group, and Christiansen/Cummings Associates. (1999). *Gambling impact and behavior study: Report to the National Gambling Impact Study Commission* [online] Available: www.norc.uchicago.edu.

Pasternak, A. V., & Fleming, M. F. (1999). Prevalence of gambling disorders in a primary care setting. *Archives of Family Medicine, 8,* 515–520.

Pavalko, R. M. (1999). Problem gambling: The hidden addiction. *National Forum, 79,* 28–32.

Pavalko, R. M. (2000). *Risky business: America's fascination with gambling.* Belmont, CA: Wadsworth.

Preston, F. W., & Smith, R. W. (1985). Delabeling and relabeling in Gamblers Anonymous: Problems with transferring the Alcoholics Anonymous paradigm. *Journal of Gambling Behavior, 1,* 185–187.

Rosecrance, J. (1988). *Gambling without guilt.* Pacific Grove, CA: Brooks/Cole.

Rosenthal, R. J. (1989). Pathological gambling and problem gambling: Problems of definition and diagnosis. In H. J. Shaffer, S. A. Stein, B. Gambino, & T. N. Cummings (Editors), *Compulsive gambling: Theory, research, and practice.* Lexington, MA: Lexington Books.

Rosenthal, R. J., & Lesieur, H. R. (1992). Self-reported withdrawal symptoms and pathological gambling. *American Journal of Addictions, 1,* 150–154.

Shaffer, H. J., Hall, M. N., & Vander Bilt, J. (1997). *Estimating the prevalence of disordered gambling behavior in the United States and Canada: A meta-analysis.* Cambridge, MA: Harvard Medical School.

Schaler, J. A. (2000). *Addiction is a choice.* Peru, IL: Open Court Publishing Company.

12

Prevention of Alcohol and Substance Misuse: Lessons for the Practitioner From a Statewide Program in Virginia

Constance L. Coogle and Nancy J. Osgood

Introduction

Although it is not widely recognized, alcohol and prescription drug abuse may affect up to 17% of elders. The gerontological and substance abuse literature both lack sufficient substantive research that addresses this neglected issue, although there are several reasons for this omission. Health care providers often mistake the symptoms of substance abuse for those of depression or dementia, while older adults are more prone to hide their disorders, and less likely to seek the help of a professional. Although it was once presumed that older adults only abused alcohol, the abuse and misuse of other drugs, especially prescription and over-the-counter medications, has begun to receive overdue recognition. Benzodiazepines, other sedatives and hypnotics, and antihistamines are commonly overprescribed, overused, or simply mismanaged.

Ageism, clinician behavior, lack of awareness, and comorbidity are all barriers to the identification and treatment of substance abuse disorders in the older population. Clinicians may be slow to spot an older individual with a substance abuse problem, and several of the DSM-IV criteria for substance abuse may not be directly applicable to the older population. Providers may also presume that older individuals do not benefit from treatment as much as younger individuals, although research shows that they are more likely to comply with treatment protocols. Comorbidity with other problems is also a barrier to diagnosing and treating substance abuse in elders. Often, elders experience an array of medical conditions including cognitive impairment, mental disorders, sensory problems, and lack of mobility which prevent or complicate a differential diagnosis. Although it is important to realize that substance abuse in the older population extends beyond problems related to alcohol abuse and alcoholism, that is the focus of this chapter.

Alcoholism is a major public health problem. *Healthy People 2010* is the current disease prevention and health promotion agenda for the nation. Focus Area 26 calls for a reduction in substance abuse. Similarly, the Public Health Service in its 1990 Health Objectives for the Nation, which were incorporated into *Healthy People 2000,* focused on the importance of health promotion and included strategies for reducing specific life-style risk factors, such as the misuse of alcohol and drugs.

The traditional model of prevention, the Public Health Model (PHM), has been applied to a wide range of medical, mental health, and human services problems and interventions. The PHM is a blended view that identifies three levels of prevention: tertiary, secondary, and primary. Tertiary prevention focuses on individuals who already display serious disorder. It includes rehabilitation, treatment, and maintenance. Secondary prevention targets individuals who demonstrate early signs of a disorder. The goal of secondary prevention is to reduce the intensity, severity, and duration of symptoms. Dr. Michael Fleming's chapter, "Identification and Treatment of Alcohol Use Disorders in Older Adults" in this volume, discusses the efficacy of brief intervention therapy (Project GOAL) as a secondary prevention strategy in older adults, and provides a detailed outline of the strategies that can be used by clinicians to motivate their patients. Guidelines for conducting these sessions with older adults have been issued as well (Center for Substance Abuse Treatment, 1998). In contrast, primary prevention aims to reduce the incidence of new cases of a disorder. Yet, there are a number of complexities involved in distinguishing between the various levels of prevention given in the traditional Public Health Model. For example, when brief intervention targets at-risk drinkers who do not yet manifest alcohol-related problems, it constitutes a primary prevention strategy that focuses on individuals in clinical settings. This therapeutic approach, then, is essentially an educational strategy aimed at health promotion and disease prevention.

The PHM also reflects a linear view of disorders as they evolve sequentially from onset through clinical syndrome (Silverman & Felner, 1995). Silverman and Felner (1995) recently pointed out that:

> to develop the precision necessary for a science of prevention, a fundamental shift must occur in our language in which we abandon the traditional public health phraseology and employ terms that are more descriptive and conceptually suited to the approaches being implemented. Adopting this perspective, tertiary prevention becomes treatment, secondary prevention becomes early intervention, and primary prevention assumes the sole mantle of prevention (p. 73).

The approach described by Silverman and Felner is referred to in the prevention literature as a unique approach in which prevention is clearly distinguished from intervention and treatment. Silverman and Felner (1995) identify four distinguishing features of prevention:

> (1) prevention occurs before the onset of illness or disorder; (2) prevention efforts are mass or population focused, rather than targeted to individuals who demonstrate signs and symptoms of some disorder; (3) prevention activities will be applied to the enhancement, disruption, or modification, as appropriate, of the unfolding process (and conditions) that lead to well-being or serious mental health or social problems; and (4) integral to prevention programming are efforts to promote strengths, well-being, and positive developmental outcomes (pp. 74–75).

The authors equate prevention with health promotion, but recent approaches include disease preventions as well.

The ultimate goal of public health is the prevention of physical diseases and mental disorders. In 1990, the Secretary of Health and Human Services named prevention as our country's number one health priority for the coming decade. Prevention has become a major priority on the public health agenda because we now recognize that interventions and treatment programs that occur after the fact are not adequate to reduce the health problems in our country. In 1991, the United Nations proposed a set of Principles for Older Persons, which emphasized wellness and health promotion through assuring independence, participation, care, self-fulfillment, and dignity.

Today, the public health approach places greater priority on health promotion and emphasizes health education and environmental support. Education is a cornerstone in disease prevention and health promotion. In *Health Promotion and Aging,* David Haber (1994) emphasizes the role of information and education in health promotion for older adults. As Haber points out, information and education can help reduce negative life-style risk factors such as smoking, alcohol abuse, and drug abuse, and help increase life-enhancing factors such as healthy eating habits and exercise patterns.

To date, very few programs focus on the primary prevention of alcoholism in older people. The statewide program in Virginia described in this chapter was designed to be such a model initiative. One major aim of the project was to prevent alcohol abuse among older adults through providing information and education to older people, caregivers of older adults, and service providers who serve older people. Another aim of the project was to enhance health and wellness in older people, and increase knowledge and information and cross-referrals in service providers who work with older people. Realizing that evaluation is a critical element in prevention programs, careful documentation of the program's impact and success was also an important project goal.

Measuring the Effectiveness of Prevention Efforts

The Need for Improved Prevention Designs and Evaluation

Just as the cost effectiveness of substance abuse treatment has been explored in order to determine financially prudent ways to serve clients (e.g., see Zarkin, French, Anderson, & Bradley, 1994) and justify the treatment dollars spent, prevention efforts must also begin responding to the increased demand for accountability (Kim, Coletti, Crutchfield, Williams, & Hepler, 1995). Health services research is critical in realizing prevention's potential to reduce the demand for future health care. In 1997, the Subcommittee on Health Services Research, National Advisory Council on Alcohol Abuse and Alcoholism, National Institute on Alcohol Abuse and Alcoholism (NIAAA) called for research that measures the effectiveness of alcohol prevention in reducing the utilization of health care services, as well as the assessment of prevention results among populations having a high level of health care services use or at risk for high-cost care. Adequate documentation of the outcomes related to educational interventions designed to prevent alcohol and substance misuse in older adults is a necessary first step. But the application of age-appropriate evaluation instruments that measure reduced consumption, decreased incidence of disease, and other harm reduction effects (e.g., preventing falls and driving accidents), should then be accompanied by investigations into the cost-savings of associated changes in the demand for health care.

The training of health care professionals and other service providers who work with older adults may be one of the most efficient means for accomplishing widespread substance abuse prevention. Yet only a few of the initiatives designed to enhance detection and prevent the misuse of alcohol and substance abuse in older adults have attempted to document the consequences of training in terms of the effect on practice (e.g., Peressini & McDonald, 1998). Even fewer have investigated the long-term impact of their interventions. Although most programs conduct some kind of short-term evaluation (same day or within a few weeks) and demonstrate gains in knowledge or attitude changes among participants, the extent to which this new knowledge improves clinical proficiency or becomes translated into ameliorative action remains undetermined. Prevention specialists need to consider how to assess workplace-based outcomes when programs are first conceived, and there are multiple advantages when a follow-up component is built into the design of these efforts.

Examples From Related Efforts

Given the lack of examples in the prevention literature specific to conducting long-term follow-up with older adults, it is instructive to look at the ways in which the effects of treatment have been documented. Many of the questions about the treatment of substance abuse problems can also be asked about programs and services that are designed to prevent those problems. The best strategies have been developed to track clients whose life situations frequently change (juveniles, the homeless, and those involved with the criminal justice system). The formative evaluation of an 18-month follow-up study in St. Louis funded by the National Institute on Drug Abuse highlighted the importance of a comprehensive tracking system, persistence, and creative teamwork (Cottler, Compton, Ben-Adallah, Horne, & Claverie, 1996). The 10 procedures to ensure effective follow-up, offered by Desmond, Maddux, Johnson, and Confer (1995) on the basis of an extensive review of the literature, are also informative.

The generic (not elder-specific) prevention literature does offer some suggestions for evaluating the effects of programs that are intended to proactively address the problem of substance abuse. The Center for Substance Abuse Prevention (CSAP) has developed a comprehensive *Guide for Evaluating Prevention Effectiveness* that provides the fundamental concepts and tools for designing and implementing successful evaluation efforts (CSAP, 1998). The Guide emphasizes the importance of collaboration between evaluators and practitioners (including administrators, program planners, and support staff) in the management of process and outcome evaluations. This advice has implications for efforts that are targeted to older adults as well. It is important to remember, however, that although methodologies can be borrowed from alcohol prevention efforts with other age groups, their applicability to older adults must be carefully considered and modified when appropriate. On the other hand, some of the lessons learned are particularly relevant to programs that target those who provide services to the older population. It has been suggested that successful prevention programs should focus not only on the individual, but also the broader environment within which the substance abuse occurs (Yin, 1993). This distinction between program-oriented and community-oriented prevention efforts is particularly significant in statewide efforts when the effect on systems is of interest. Beyond assessing the impact of an individual's participation in a program, assessment should also focus on the extent to which programs result in lasting improvements in the way services are delivered. Yin (1993) suggests that the formative evaluation of a single education program can entail multiple study designs that not only document the service intervention in terms of client outcomes, but also examine how interagency and community processes (as well as empowerment and family dynamics) affect their associated outcomes.

Beyond the theoretical advice, there has been some practice-based direction that has relevance for prevention in older adults (Aguirre-Molina & Gorman, 1996). Literature reviews have summarized what is known about community-based substance abuse prevention programs, and how they can best be evaluated (Gorman & Speer, 1996). But educational programs that have targeted service providers are more directly related to the possibility of producing improvements in the detection and prevention of substance abuse. It would be wise, therefore, to design prevention and evaluation strategies on the basis of more generalized PHMs. Some emergent foundational principles, recently offered by those working in the area of alcohol and aging, should be considered as well.

Emerging Examples of Elder-Specific Evaluation Models

It has been stipulated that there are no rigorously randomized prevention studies focusing on the elderly, and that there is inadequate basic research to support full-scale intervention trials (Boyd, 1998). To the extent that this is the case, the situation may likely be temporary. The Center for Substance Abuse Prevention (CSAP) has recently instituted the Community Initiated Prevention Intervention program which provides funding for the development of innovative substance abuse prevention interventions. Although the initiative is not specifically targeted to gerontologists, the American Society on Aging was included in the first cohort of cooperative agreements awarded. The "Aging and Alcohol Community-Based Brief Intervention Project" is employing NIAAA standards for selecting at-risk elders who are randomly assigned to an intervention or control group. The project serves as a concrete example of using brief intervention as a primary prevention strategy. CSAP has also developed the National Registry of Effective Prevention Programs (NREPP) which reviews formally evaluated prevention initiatives using a formal peer review process and a standardized 15–criteria protocol to identify model and promising programs. The NREPP has identified one model program with an intergenerational focus, and is in the process of reviewing additional programs aimed at older adults.

Recent Guidance Offered

In addition to the instructive examples found in the few models that have emerged, there is also a general understanding about the theoretical issues that should be considered when developing the evaluation of such interventions. Although there are a number of questions about the optimal delivery format and content of the prevention message to older populations, program planners cannot wait for the definitive answers. Evaluation efforts must also proceed, and there are some conceptual issues that provide guidance in this area. Variation in the definitions used to ascribe different age groups, life-course changes in drinking habits, and differences in the risk profiles for specific subpopulations must all be considered (Gomberg, Hegedus, & Zucker, 1998). Prevention objectives should also not be limited to simple intake reduction or control. The definition of abusive drinking needs to be adjusted as circumstances differ, as for example when medication interactions are involved. Gomberg and colleagues (1998) have proposed that there is a spectrum of limits for problem use that varies with age and medical circumstance analogous to Blow's (1998) spectrum of interventions (Gomberg et al., 1998). This proposition should be pursued.

The Statewide Program in Virginia: Detection and Prevention

Virginia was the first state in the country to conduct a statewide detection and primary prevention program for geriatric alcoholism. The effort targeted older adults, their families, their caregivers, and professionals in the fields of aging, medicine, and mental health about alcoholism in the elderly. This initiative serves as a model of how alcohol prevention programs can be successfully implemented and evaluated.

Coalition-Building

One aim of the project was to bring together individuals from different agencies and backgrounds, including health, mental health, substance abuse, and aging, to network, share ideas and information, and work together. We wanted participants to get to know each other personally and become familiar with the wide range of different services available to older individuals at risk for developing alcohol problems. The hope was that by building strong coalitions, we would increase information sharing and referrals between agencies.

The first step we took to build coalitions was to form an Advisory Committee that would be involved in every step of the project from choosing the primary trainer, to recruiting volunteer trainers, to designing the evaluation instrument. The Advisory Committee included individuals from the Virginia Department of Health, the Virginia Department for the Aging, the Virginia Department of Mental Health, Mental Retardation, and Substance Abuse Services, the Virginia Department of Social Services, Alcoholics Anonymous, and the American Association of Retired Persons, as well as individuals from local community service boards and area agencies on aging and physicians. The Advisory Committee met regularly throughout the project.

The next step we took was to develop a list of all volunteer trainers with addresses and phone numbers. We mailed the list to all trainers so that they could identify the other trainers in their region and perhaps contact them. Shortly after mailing out the list of trainers, we held an all-day satellite videoconference on alcoholism and aging in each region of the state (Coogle, Osgood, Parham, Wood, & Churcher, 1995). This was the first event that brought volunteer trainers in each region together to meet each other.

The next coalition-building event we had was the all-day training session for volunteer trainers. Trainers from each region were brought together in a location in their region to attend an all-day training session conducted by a professional trainer. At this event trainers socialized and learned valuable information together. At the end of the day, volunteer trainers were paired into training teams. We specifically teamed individuals from different agencies. For example, a service worker from a mental health agency was teamed with a service provider from an aging agency. The two-person teams shared information and worked together to conduct training sessions in their region. The purpose of teaming individuals from different services and agencies was to assure that people in different agencies got to meet one another and work together, shared information with one another, and became familiar with different services offered in other agencies that serve older people in their region. An additional reason for teaming in this way was to increase cross-referrals between different types of agencies and services.

Developing and Providing Good Quality Information

Another goal of the Statewide Program in Virginia was to develop and provide good quality information on alcoholism and aging and on services available to help older individuals with alcohol problems. At the time the project received funding, there was a lack of good quality, easy-to-understand information on the topic available. Information was provided to volunteer trainers through the satellite teleconference and an all-day training session conducted by a professional trainer. In addition, volunteer trainers were given additional informational pamphlets and brochures and a list of references on the topic. The Statewide Program in Virginia also produced four informational products appropriate for service providers, care givers, and older adults themselves: a community service directory of all health, mental health, aging, and substance abuse services available in each region of the state with addresses and phone numbers; a 13-minute color video; a small brochure; and a 16-page booklet. The brochure developed for the project was adapted for use with Hispanic and Asian (Japanese-speaking) populations, the focus was expanded to encompass any kind of substance abuse, and outreach to the African American community was implemented with state-level funding. A master Replication Plan created for the project guided continued education and outreach efforts throughout the Commonwealth.

Organizing and Overseeing Statewide Training

One major goal of the project was to train a large number of service providers, care givers, and older adults across the state. To reach this goal, teams of volunteer trainers conducted training sessions in their local communities in each region of the state. Volunteer trainers were recruited with the help of members of the Advisory Committee through newsletters and other publications, by word of mouth, and through a variety of other techniques. Volunteer trainers were very well trained before conducting their training sessions. They were given a standardized training curriculum to use to conduct their training sessions to assure standardized training across the state. In the all-day training sessions, volunteer trainers were trained in how to recruit for and publicize sessions in their local area. They had the opportunity to meet individuals from area agencies on aging, community service boards, and other agencies in their region. Individuals from these agencies agreed to help trainers recruit people for training sessions and to provide space and a television/VCR when needed. The project included a person whose main job responsibilities included working with volunteer trainers and tracking the training across the state. This individual helped set up training sessions for some trainers. She kept in regular contact with all trainers by phone, cards, and mail. One of her responsibilities was to encourage trainers. Members of the project staff also attended parties at the homes of trainers, appeared on television programs organized by volunteer trainers, and tried to remain intimately involved with trainers throughout the project.

Evaluating Effectiveness

To judge the effectiveness of training and training materials, evaluation is essential. Both short-term and long-term effects of training should be evaluated. To evaluate the short-term effects of training, we developed and administered a pretest and posttest of knowledge about alcoholism and aging to all volunteer trainers and all individuals trained in the short training sessions in the local community. We also administered the knowledge questionnaire to a small control group. Statistical analyses of data revealed that the training was very effective. Subsequent interviews with agency personnel revealed a substantive impact on a broad spectrum of service systems, as well as improvements in interagency coordination (Coogle, Osgood, & Parham, 2000a; Coogle, Osgood, Pyles, & Wood, 1995).

A follow-up study was conducted to investigate the long-term consequences of the statewide geriatric alcoholism detection and primary prevention effort in Virginia. High levels of knowledge had been retained seven years after the initial training. The results of this study are given elsewhere (Coogle, Osgood, & Parham, in press) and summarized in Table 12.1. Quantitative and qualitative data, provided by almost half of the volunteers who were trained to conduct workshops in their communities, verified the program's ability to: 1) promote information-sharing with others, 2) enhance the detection of alcohol problems, and 3) increase the incidence of assistance to individuals with alcohol problems. The study also provided evidence that participation in the project stimulated further training or study in the area of geriatric substance abuse, and results from the follow-up knowledge test verified that learning had been retained over time. The training sessions were successful in sending a personal message about alcoholism, as well as a professional one. Although the program was not designed to change the personal drinking habits of the participants, 10% of respondents said that participation had caused them to reduce their consumption, and almost as many had quit drinking altogether.

Composite Case Illustrating Intervention Effectiveness

The case which follows is a composite based on the results of short- and long-term evaluation of the statewide program in Virginia. Although

Table 12.1. Long-Term Follow-Up of Community Trainers

Usefulness of Participation
- Training Day Very Useful (69%)
- Booklet, Brochure, & Video Very Useful (> 50%)
- Community Services Directory
  - * Moderately/Very Useful (69%)
  - * Used to Help Clients (36.5%)

Program Resulted in Information Dissemination
- 70% shared information with clients
- 85% with professional colleagues
- 22% with family member with drinking problem
- 40% with other family member
- 62% with someone else

Identification and Referral Attributed to Training
- 71% applied information to detect alcohol problems
- 62% encouraged participation in 12–step program
- 75% encouraged help-seeking behavior

Program Encouraged Assistance to Others
- Training greatly/moderately improved ability to assist with alcohol problem (> 75%)
- Training greatly increased likelihood of taking action when encountering an older person who might have a problem with alcohol (about 50%)

Program Stimulated Further Training or Study
- 95% independently studied geriatric alcoholism
- 44% participated in geriatric alcoholism training
- 44% participated in further training related to general field of alcoholism/substance abuse
- 46% participated in aging-related training

Program Influenced Personal Drinking Habits of Participants
- 10% reduced their alcohol consumption
- 5% eliminated their alcohol consumption
- 8% indicated that training aided their recovery

Sarah M. and Mrs. P. are fictional characters, their experiences are drawn from qualitative and quantitative feedback provided by those who actually participated as trainers in the project.

> Sarah M., a licensed clinical social worker, recently assumed the position of Adult Services Program Manager in the central office of the State Department of Social Services (DSS). As she settled into the new position she began to realize that substance abuse issues were beginning to surface in several of the programs. Local preadmission screening profiles, the statewide

uniform information monitoring system interviews, assessments of adult care residents across the state, and reports from the home-based service providers all included a surprising number of cases where substance abuse was either contributing to existing problems or constituting an additional problem that deserved attention. Although case managers at the local social services offices verbally supported what Sarah was seeing in the paperwork, they were not particularly alarmed. They were, to some extent, amused when encountering these "sweet" clients who were trying to stay "young at heart" by "continuing to enjoy one of the few pleasures left in their lives." Some commented that older adults with lifelong drinking histories "are too old to change their habits now." Others who had encountered elders with alcohol-related brain disease claimed that, "these people are so far gone there isn't much you can say to reach them." Even members of her own staff made off-hand comments about how "these poor old people should be able to do something to lift their spirits."

When the Geriatric Education Center produced a teleconference on geriatric alcoholism, Sarah encouraged her staff to attend. Then, when the University and the State Unit on Aging collaborated to implement a statewide train-the-trainer program, Sarah made sure that select personnel at the local offices registered for the all-day training sessions in their localities. She participated on the state level Steering Committee, and assisted with the recruitment of older adults at risk and their family members. The trainer fliers were distributed through the local offices, and social workers in the individual localities posted the fliers in nontraditional locations such as community bulletin boards. Most of the DSS personnel who attended the training partnered with case managers they met from the local Area Agencies on Aging, and proceeded to provide workshops in their communities. Sarah knew that her efforts had been worthwhile when someone on her staff confided that the training "helped me to be more tolerant and compassionate toward the clients who may be experiencing substance abuse problems."

Because of Sarah's participation on the Steering Committee, the Department of Social Services was able to develop linkages with the State Unit on Aging and the Department of Mental Health/Substance Abuse Services. At the regional and local levels, those who were trained began to form more collaborative relationships with other agencies. By using the Community Resources Directory provided in the training, interagency referrals and case consultations increased. Systemwide, it seemed that the coordination of services delivered to older adults at risk had been enhanced.

Sarah inquired at the local DSS offices whether there had been any improvement in the detection of the signs and symptoms of alcohol abuse in the field. She discovered that evidence of falling accidents or unstable gait that might have been simply attributed to age-related illness prior to the training, was now being investigated more systematically as a consequence of increased awareness. Social workers were making more referrals to the local mental health center when substance abuse became recognized, and some were making transportation arrangements for clients to attend Alcoholic Anonymous meetings during the day (the preferred time for many older adults). Clients, who may have taken up drinking because of social isolation or loss, were being connected with senior centers and encouraged to find opportunities to volunteer.

One particularly revealing case involved an encounter with a 70–year-old widow, Mrs. P., who habitually drank a glass of wine with dinner just as she and her deceased husband had done when they were younger. Lately, she had continued to have another glass or two while watching her favorite evening game show, and sometimes another, when she had trouble falling asleep at night. Mrs. P. confided in the social worker that she had been experiencing headaches and dizziness. Mrs. P. wondered if it could be related to the wine, although she insisted, "I've never had anything like a hangover." The social worker consulted with a geropsychiatric nurse practitioner she had been partnered with during the training project. Together they determined that Mrs. P. had uncontrolled high blood pressure, and advised her to get an appointment with her family doctor. The social worker also explained to Mrs. P. that extended and regular consumption of alcohol might have contributed to her high blood pressure and advised her to quit drinking immediately. During a subsequent visit the social worker discovered that Mrs. P. had been prescribed propranolol (Inderal®) to treat her high blood pressure, but was still taking her daily glass of wine. Mrs. P. explained that her doctor had cautioned her about having more than one drink each day, but had also discussed the beneficial effects of moderate alcohol consumption on the cardiovascular system. The social worker told Mrs. P. that chronic alcohol consumption decreases the availability of propranolol, potentially reducing its therapeutic effect. She then got the name of Mrs. P.'s doctor and, by presenting herself as a patient advocate for Mrs. P., proceeded to set up a consultation. The social worker was permitted to have a long discussion with the physician and attempted to impress upon him the importance of eliminating all alcohol for his at-risk patients taking blood pressure medicine.

This particular social worker came to be regarded by her coworkers as the person to consult whenever substance abuse arose as a potential issue among their clients. Sarah M. found that the same was true in other local offices. When trainers returned to their workplaces and held seminars for their colleagues, they became regarded as the trusted and accessible resident expert.

Sarah M. always remembered her accomplishments as a leader in this statewide project. She had recognized a need to improve the state of awareness regarding treatment options for older adults with substance abuse problems, and was able to do something about it. As she observed the changes in her own agency and other departments around the state, she was gratified that she had been such an important agent for change in this worthwhile endeavor. Many years later, she talked with some of the university faculty who had received the original project grant funding from the U.S. Administration on Aging. The project directors were especially touched by reports from recovering alcoholics who had volunteered to be trainers. They told Sarah about how involvement in the project had affected the sobriety of these former alcoholics. Several of the participants continued to have renewed empathy and compassion for the older newcomers who connect with their 12–step programs. Others emphasized the significance of their realization that the detrimental effects of alcohol can be much more serious in older adults. As one put it, "Should I relapse as I grow older, the greater harm [there will be] to myself."

Implications of Related Model Projects

Other projects have also developed effective prevention programs that incorporate elements such as effective coalition building and practice-based training. Each program has faced issues of cost-effectiveness and other economic considerations. Some of these projects are summarized in Table 12.2.

Economic Considerations

Education is the key to primary prevention. But education creates the need for further and expanded information. With increased awareness comes a proportional increase in the demand for additional (perhaps specialized) treatment and recovery programs, and there are other expense demands associated with the prevention initiatives as well. Compulsory continuing education would assure that information gets to the providers who are least knowledgeable and interested in the subject. It would not only enhance the effectiveness of preventive education, but improve the process of evaluation as well. If the self-selecting bias can be excluded as a threat to validity through the institution of mandated training, some of the limitations that now hamper the conclusions drawn from evaluation efforts would be lifted.

Alternative educational models that would facilitate the translation of

Table 12.2 Other Primary Prevention Efforts

Program	Coalition-Building Efforts	Practice-Based Implications	Economic Considerations
American Society on Aging (Cullinane, 1998)	Need assessment results pointed to advantages when service agencies work collaboratively	Community-wide training and agency-specific technical assistance offered	Requests typically exceed budgetary capacity, although innovative problem-solving has extended initiative
Michigan Older Adult Substance Abuse Network[a]	Strengthen collaborative working relationships between state and local organizations	Established Leadership Council to serve as a resource for technical assistance and support to providers	Promoted increased awareness among policy makers and general public
NCoA/SAMHSA Initiative[a]	Aim to encourage more successful collaboration between service networks and community linkages for advocacy	Convened telefocus and work groups of service providers and community activists to guide content of Turnkey Kit	Financing services for older adults was third important area of recommendations
Texas Interagency Seniors and Substance Abuse Workgroup[a]	Establish Memorandum of Understanding to promote coordinated service delivery	Action plan and specific strategies for expanding treatment options	Seeks to identify and maximize existing resources
Virginia Institute of Social Services Training Activities (Teitelman & O'Neill, 1998)	Statewide advisory group develops competency-based curriculum	Attitudinal and behavioral intention changes documented	Concerned that mandates for training of service providers are viewed as cost-prohibitive
Wisconsin Coalition on Mental Health/Substance Abuse/Aging[a]	Emphasis on local collaborative support	Developed age-appropriate services	When grant ended, advocacy efforts led to ongoing support with county funds

[a]Contact information related to these projects is given in the Promising Practices Nominations workbook, NCoA, (202) 479–6671

instruction into practice are justified, but securing the needed funding is a challenge. In addition, any expanded evaluation effort to document the practice-based outcomes of training will require increased funding appropriations. Without sufficient funding, educational interventions can easily result in a frustrated infrastructure that is incapable of supporting the need for services. One encouraging long-term evaluation, however, suggests that outreach and identification does not necessarily result in increased service utilization and greater burden on the service system. Those involved in the Community Gatekeeper Model project have demonstrated that clients who are referred through their initiative are no more likely than those referred through other sources to be placed out of home one year after their initial identification (Florio, Jensen, Hendryx, Raschko, & Mathieson, 1998). To the contrary, results suggest that they may have an enhanced ability to continue living in the community. In fact, the model is inexpensive to implement and can benefit communities through increased collaboration among service providers. As was discussed in the beginning of this chapter, it is time to conduct some comprehensive cost-benefit analyses to reinforce the argument for adequate funding. It would be advantageous to document the cost-savings associated with the implementation of successful prevention efforts, as well as expanded treatment programs resulting as a consequence of improved identification and awareness. Unfortunately, there are methodological issues that complicate these kinds of evaluations, and the lack of research in this area is particularly frustrating now that questions about program effectiveness are being linked increasingly with questions about program costs (see Werthamer & Chatterji, 1998 for a review of the literature). There are difficulties related to assigning costs to intervention and comparison conditions, and there are problems in measuring outcomes that do not occur generally until many years after a program's completion. These two critical challenges must be met before policy makers become convinced to devote proportionate public dollars to prevention research and initiatives.

Recommendations for Future Efforts

The project in Virginia was the first statewide education and training program on geriatric alcoholism conducted in the country. It has served as a model for other projects. Table 12.3 lists some of the important

Table 12.3 Lessons Learned From the Statewide Program in Virginia

- A news story in the local paper is helpful to make the public aware of the issue. An Associated Press story on the project and the trainers reaches an even larger audience.
- Reach hard-to-reach communities such as minorities by involving them on the Advisory Committee and selecting training sites conducive to their participation.
- Allow for plenty of staff to organize, plan, track, and follow-up with trainers. Hiring graduate students can often maximize limited resources.
- Improve your own networking by nominating a key player in a nonaging field for an aging-related award or issue them a certificate of appreciation from your Advisory Committee.
- Work your project plans into the official or strategic plan of the State Unit on Aging or the Mental Health Department. This provides a continuing basis for advocacy on behalf of your project.
- Review the qualifications of potential trainers with some of the key players. Soliciting their involvement will help ensure a quality selection process and strengthen their commitment to the project.
- Use health facilities, inpatient treatment facilities, and offices of local service providers for the training. This reduces costs and helps to reach the substance abuse service network.
- Give CEU's for any major training sessions held. The added benefit will improve the response to training.
- Keep the volunteer trainers involved and informed with a personal touch by sending them regular updates and information and greeting cards at major holiday times.
- Use newsletters of as wide a variety of groups as possible as a source of recruitment and publicity.
- Many information and referral centers have sophisticated database search capabilities. A listing which cross references aging and substance abuse may become the core of your service directory.
- Use a graphic and verbal theme or motif to connect the publications of the project.
- Videotape key events and training conducted so that future trainers can view them and receive the same orientation.
- If funding is obtained, write letters of understanding with grant coparticipants and key players to clearly specify the roles of each.

lessons learned and provides tips that should help others develop a successful education and training effort in their state or local community. In addition, study of the Virginia project and related initiatives has given rise to recommendations for future efforts. Those who would implement prevention programs to address substance abuse problems in older adults are advised to consider:

(a) implementing a competency-based or systemwide needs assessment prior to commencement;
(b) planning both short- and long-term outcome evaluation studies that include a cost effectiveness component, examine workplace-based outcomes, and employ age-appropriate measures;
(c) targeting the broader community, and examining outcomes related to interagency systems change as well as client-oriented outcomes;
(d) incorporating a technical assistance component to ensure quality and maintain a cadre of experts;
(e) establishing a mechanism for ongoing collaboration between substance abuse and aging service agencies; and
(f) advocating for mandated training or licensure requirements that could be fulfilled by participation in the training program.

A Call for More Prevention Education and Training

The prevention of late-life alcoholism is increasingly important as the population of older adults continues to grow. Future cohorts of older adults, who did not experience Prohibition and who were involved in the Vietnam War and the drug culture of the 1960s, will likely have more significant drug and alcohol problems than the current generation of elders. Education efforts to reduce biases held by health and social care providers and promote more vigilant screening may be our most significant weapon in the fight against the impending epidemiological trend. In addition, older adults, family members, and other informal caregivers also need to be better informed. Recently widowed men, older men with a history of depression or suicidal behavior, and others who are lonely and isolated, are prime targets for outreach and education programs (Osgood, Wood, & Parham, 1995). If we can surmount the barriers that have produced a general failure to inquire about alcohol-related history and habits, we may have a chance to curtail a pattern of habitual drinking before it becomes a well-established lifestyle indicator.

Acknowledgment

The Statewide Program in Virginia was supported, in part, by award number 90AM0389–91 from the Administration on Aging, Department of Health and Human Services, Washington, DC 20201.

References

Aguirre-Molina, M., & Gorman, D. M. (1996). Community-based approaches for the prevention of alcohol, tobacco, and other drug use. *Annual Review of Public Health, 17,* 337–358.

Blow, F. C. (1998). The spectrum of alcohol interventions for older adults. In E. S. L. Gomberg, A. M. Hegedus, & R. A. Zucker (Editors), *Alcohol problems and aging* (Research Monograph No. 33) (pp. 373–396). Bethesda, MD: National Institute on Alcohol Abuse and Alcoholism.

Boyd, G. M. (1998). Commentary on prevention of alcohol problems in the elderly. In E. S. L. Gomberg, A. M. Hegedus, & R. A. Zucker (Editors), *Alcohol problems and aging* (Research Monograph No. 33) (pp. 439–447). Bethesda, MD: National Institute on Alcohol Abuse and Alcoholism.

Center for Substance Abuse Prevention. (1998). *A guide for evaluating prevention effectiveness.* (CSAP Publication No. SMA 98–3237). Rockville, MD: USDHHS, PHS, & SAMHSA.

Center for Substance Abuse Treatment. (1998). *Substance abuse among older adults.* Treatment Improvement Protocol (TIP) Series, No. 26. (CSAT Publication No. SMA 98–3179). Rockville, MD: USDHHS, PHS, & SAMHSA.

Coogle, C. L., Osgood, N. O., & Parham, I. A. (2000a). A statewide model detection and prevention program for geriatric alcoholism and alcohol abuse: Increased knowledge among service providers. *Community Mental Health Journal, 36*(2), 137–148.

Coogle, C. L., Osgood, N. O., & Parham, I. A. (in press). Follow-up to the statewide model detection and prevention program for geriatric alcoholism and alcohol abuse. *Community Mental Health Journal.*

Coogle, C. L., Osgood, N. J., Parham, I. A., Wood, H. E., & Churcher, C. S. (1995). The effectiveness of videoconferencing in geriatric alcoholism education. *Gerontology and Geriatrics Education, 16*(2), 73–83.

Coogle, C. L., Osgood, N. J., Pyles, M. A., & Wood, H. E. (1995). The impact of alcoholism education on service providers, elders, and their family members. *Journal of Applied Gerontology, 14*(3), 321–332.

Cottler, L. L., Compton, W., Ben-Adallah, A., Horne, M., & Claverie, D. (1996). Achieving a 96.6% follow-up rate in a longitudinal study of drug abusers. *Drug and Alcohol Dependence, 41,* 209–217.

Cullinane, P. C. (1998). A statewide project to increase accessibility of older adults to substance abuse services. *The Southwest Journal on Aging, 14*(1), 19–26.

Desmond, D. P., Maddux, J. F., Johnson, T. H., & Confer, B. A. (1995). Obtaining follow-up interviews for treatment evaluation. *Journal of Substance Abuse Treatment, 12,* 95–102.

Florio, E. R., Jensen, J. E., Hendryx, M., Raschko, R., & Mathieson, K. (1998).

One-year outcomes of older adults referred for aging and mental health services by community gatekeepers. *Journal of Case Management, 7*(2), 74–83.

Gomberg, E. S. L., Hegedus, A. M., & Zucker. R. A. (1998). Research issues and priorities. In E. S. L. Gomberg, A. M. Hegedus, & R. A. Zucker (Editors), *Alcohol problems and aging* (Research Monograph No. 33) (pp. 452–475). Bethesda, MD: National Institute on Alcohol Abuse and Alcoholism.

Gorman, D. M., & Speer, P. W. (1996). Preventing alcohol abuse and alcohol-related problems through community interventions: A review of evaluation studies. *Psychology and Health, 11*(1), 95–131.

Haber, D. (1994). *Health promotion and aging.* New York: Springer Publishing.

Kim, S., Coletti, S. D., Crutchfield, C. C., Williams, C., & Hepler, N. (1995). Benefit-cost analysis of drug abuse prevention programs: A macroscopic approach. *Journal of Drug Education, 25*(2), 111–127.

Osgood, N. J., Wood, H. E., & Parham, I. A. (1995). *Alcoholism and aging: An annotated bibliography and review.* Westport, CT: Greenwood Press.

Peressini, T., & McDonald, L. (1998). Evaluation of a training program on alcoholism and older adults for health care and social service practitioners. *Gerontology and Geriatrics Education, 18*(4), 23–44.

Silverman, M. M., & Felner, R. D. (1995). The place of suicide prevention in the spectrum of intervention: Definitions of critical terms and constructs. *Suicide and Life-Threatening Behavior, 25*(1), 70–81.

Teitelman, J., & O'Neill, P. (1998). Alcohol and medication abuse: A statewide competency-based curriculum for adult services/adult protective service workers. *The Southwest Journal on Aging, 14*(1), 27–33.

Walker, B. L. (1998) Problem use of alcohol: A training program for long-term care staff. *The Southwest Journal on Aging, 14*(1), 35–41.

Werthamer, L., & Chatterji, P. (1998). Preventive intervention cost-effectiveness and cost benefit. [On-line]. Bethesda, MD: National Institute on Drug Abuse. Available: http://165.112.78.61/HSR/da-pre/WerthamerPreventive.htm.

Yin, R. K. (1993). Lessons learned about the effects of community-based prevention programs. In R. K. Yin (Editor), *Applications of case study research: Applied Social Research Methods Series, 34* (pp.94–108). Newbury Park, CA: Sage Publications.

Zarkin, G. A., French, M. T., Anderson, D. W., & Bradley, C. J. (1994). Conceptual framework for the economic evaluation of substance abuse interventions. *Evaluation and Program Planning, 17,* 409–418.

Index

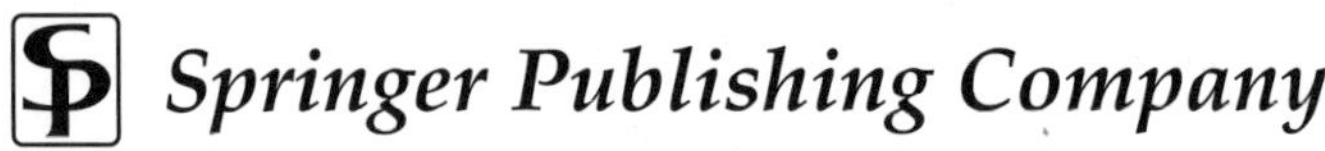

Alcohol Problems in Older Adults

Prevention and Management

Kristen Lawton Barry, PhD, **David W. Oslin,** MD, and **Frederic C. Blow,** PhD

This manual provides state-of-the-art, practical materials to detect, prevent, and intervene with older adults who are at-risk and problem drinkers. It provides the first systematic, practical approach for working in a variety of clinical settings with a growing vulnerable population of older adults who use alcohol at risk levels often unnoticed in everyday clinical practice.

It is designed as a "hands-on" document for use in primary and mental health care settings by physicians, nurse practitioners, nurses, social workers, psychologists, and case managers. Chapters include guides to alcohol screening, assessments, brief interventions, intensive care referrals, and protocols for managing withdrawal care. Dialogue examples are interwoven throughout. In addition, appendices include an English/Spanish Health Promotion Workbook for Older Adults that can be reproduced for non-commercial purposes.

Contents: Preface • **Section 1:** Introduction and Background • **Section 2:** Alcohol Screening • **Section 3:** Brief Alcohol Interventions • **Section 4:** Frequently Asked Questions • **Section 5:** Special Circumstances • **Section 6:** Community Resources • References

Appendices:

Educational Forms and Patient Handouts

Health Promotion Workbook for Older Adults:
Initial Session, English and Spanish Translations

Health Promotion Workbook for Older Adults:
Follow-up Session, English and Spanish Translations

2001 152pp 0-8261-1403-2 soft

536 Broadway, New York, NY 10012-3955 • (212) 431-4370 • Fax (212) 941-7842 Order Toll-Free: (877) 687-7476 • Order On-line: ***www.springerpub.com***

Springer Publishing Company

Older Adults' Misuse of Alcohol, Medicines, and Other Drugs

Research and Practice Issues

Anne M. Gurnack, MSW, PhD, Editor

Comprised of contributions by an internationally known multidisciplinary team of experts, this volume presents the latest thinking and research findings on alcohol and drug misuse in later life. Part I reviews the epidemiology and assessment of problem drinking. It includes a useful review of medical manifestations of alcoholism; techniques on how to detect early versus late onset of alcoholism; and treatment alternatives for alcohol abusers. Part II focuses on prescriptive and illicit drug abuse. This volume will be a resource to researchers of many disciplines including gerontology, social work, and nursing.

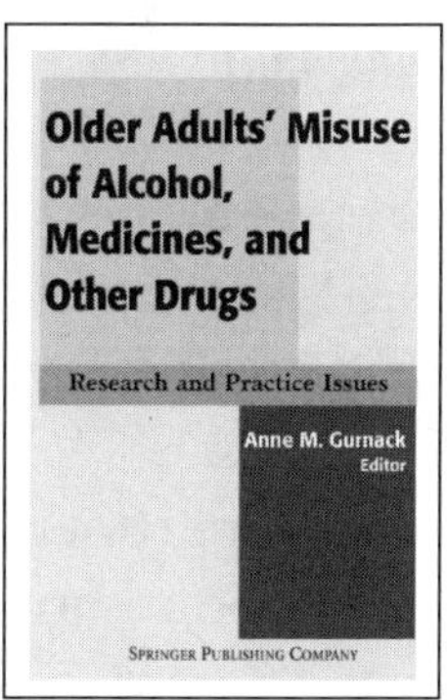

Contents:

Foreword: Edith S. Lisansky Gomberg

- Introduction, *Anne M. Gurnack*
- Epidemiology of Problem Drinking Among Elderly People, *Wendy L. Adams, MD, MPH and Narra Smith Cox, PhD*
- Screening and Diagnosis of Alcohol Use Disorders in Older Adults, *Sara S. DeHart, MSN, PhD, RN and Norman G. Hoffman, PhD*
- Medical Manifestations of Alcoholism in the Elderly, *James W. Smith*
- Early Versus Late Onset of Alcoholism in the Elderly, *Joseph G. Liberto, MD and David W. Oslin, MD*
- Treatment Alternatives for Older Alcohol Abusers, *Lawrence Schonfeld, PhD and Larry Dupree, PhD*
- Alcoholism and Dementia, *David M. Smith, MD and Roland M. Atkinson, MD*
- Misuse of Prescription Drugs, *Richard Finlayson, MD*
- Interactions Between Alcohol and Other Drugs, *Wendy L. Adams, MD, MPH*
- Illicit Drug Use and Abuse Among Older People, *Helen Rosenberg, PhD*
- Alcohol and Drug Misuse in the Nursing Home, *Carol Joseph, MD*

1996 296pp 0-8261-9500-8 hard

536 Broadway, New York, NY 10012-3955 • (212) 431-4370 • Fax (212) 941-7842 Order Toll-Free: (877) 687-7476 • Order On-line: ***www.springerpub.com***

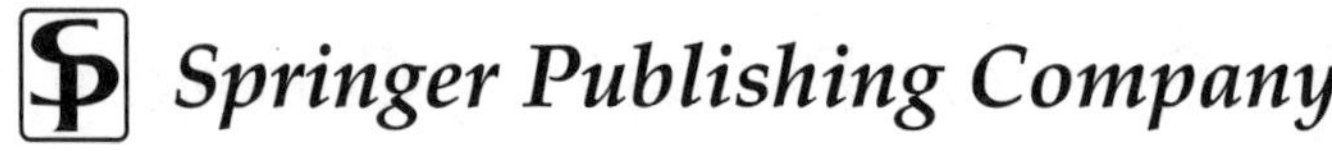

Comparative Treatments of Substance Abuse

E. Thomas Dowd, PhD and **Loreen Rugle**, PhD, Editors

"...provides important theoretical and clinical information that will be of great use to psychotherapy students...It will make an excellent companion resource to many specific chemical dependence treatment texts because it provides a variety of theories that are clearly linked to practical intervention strategies." —**George Buelow,** PhD
Department of Psychology, University of Southern Mississippi, Hattiesburg, MS

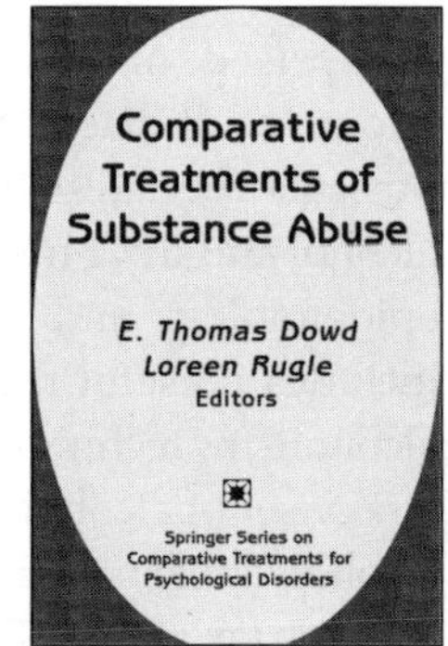

Partial Contents: Substance Abuse in American Society, *E. Thomas Dowd & Loreen G. Rugle* • Outcome Research in Substance Abuse Treatment, *Carole A. Putt* • The Case of "Paul," *Loreen G. Rugle & E. Thomas Dowd* • A Psychodynamic Approach to Treatment, *Richard Hirschman & Michael Foster* • Behavioral Systems Approach, *Douglas H. Ruben* • Cognitive Therapy of Substance Abuse, *Cory F. Newman & Christine L. Ratto* • Thinking Your Way Clean: Rational Emotive Behavior Therapy with a Poly-Substance Abuser, *Raymond DiGiuseppe & Jennifer Mascolo* • Client-Centered and Holistic Approach for Older Persons With Addiction Problems, *Kathryn Graham & Jane Baron* • Client-Driven, Research-Guided Treatment for Substance Users: Bringing Harm Reduction to Clinical Practice, *Frederick Rotgers* • Relapse Prevention and Harm Reduction in the Treatment of Co-Occurring Addiction and Mental Health Problems, *Kimberley Barrett & G. Alan Marlatt* • Family Therapy, *Helen S. Raytek* • Application of the Community Reinforcement Approach, Robert J. Meyers, *Jane Ellen Smith & V. Ann Waldorf* • The Case of Paul: A Systematic Approach to Ericksonian Utilization and Therapeutic Change, *William J. Matthews* • Comparative Treatments: Summary and Conclusion, *E. Thomas Dowd, Pamela J. Millas, and Loreen G. Rugle*

1999 304pp 0-8261-1276-5 hard

536 Broadway, New York, NY 10012-3955 • (212) 431-4370 • Fax (212) 941-7842 Order Toll-Free: (877) 687-7476 • Order On-line: ***www.springerpub.com***